PREGNENOLONE
Nature's Feel Good Hormone

RAY SAHELIAN, M.D.

Avery Publishing Group
Garden City Park, New York

Cover design: William Gonzalaz
Typesetters: William Gonzalaz and Elaine V. McCaw
In-house: editor: Lisa James
Printer: Paragon Press, Honesdale, PA

Avery Publishing Group, Inc.
120 Old Broadway
Garden City Park, New York 11040
1-800-548-5757

Cataloging-in-Publication Data

Sahelian, Ray
  Pregnenolone : nature's feel good hormome / by Ray Sahelian.
  p. cm.
  Includes bibliographical references and index.
  ISBN 0-89529-803-1

  1. Steroid hormones. 2. Steroid hormones—Therapeutic use.
  I. Title

  QP572.S7S24 1997   612.4'05
                                        QB197-508

CONTENTS

ACKNOWLEDGMENTS

Researchers

Etienne-Emile Baulieu, M.D., Ph.D., Professor, College of France, Paris, and Director of the Institut National de la Sante et de la Recherche Medicale (similar to the US NIH), Department of Hormone Research. Dr. Baulieu was kind enough to mail me galley proofs of his article submitted to *Recent Progress in Hormone Research* (volume 52, 1997) entitled *Neurosteroids: of the Nervous System, by the Nervous System, for the Nervous System.*

James F. Flood, Ph.D., from Medical Research Service, St. Louis University School of Medicine, St. Louis, Missouri, has studied the effects of Preg on memory in rodents.

Seymour Lieberman, Ph.D., St. Luke's–Roosevelt Hospital Center, New York, New York, has always, on multiple occasions, graciously taken his time to share his knowledge of his favorite topic, steroid hormones.

Maria Majewska, Ph.D., of the National Institute on Drug Abuse, Medications Development Division, Rockville, Maryland, is one of the world's foremost authorities on the

v

neurological aspects of DHEA, pregnenolone, and other steroid hormones. During my interview she reported that, unfortunately, very little research has been done on pregnenolone in humans. At this time, many researchers who work with these steroids are concentrating their efforts more on DHEA, and it will take a few years before their attention turns to pregnenolone.

John Morley, M.D., Professor of Medicine at the Division of Geriatrics in St. Louis University, St. Louis, Missouri, is currently conducting trials in administering this hormone to older individuals and evaluating memory, cognition, and other mental and physical parameters.

Eugene Roberts, M.D., of the Department of Biochemistry, Beckman Research Institute of the City of Hope, in Duarte, California. I sincerely wish to thank him for the time he took discussing pregnenolone with me. Although Dr. Roberts does not wish to be quoted from our conversations, he is very comfortable in being cited from the articles he has written. An excellent review article on pregnenolone by Dr. Roberts was written in 1995 in *Biochemical Pharmacology*, volume 49, number 1, pages 1–16. This article stimulated my interest in Preg.

Rahmawati Sih, M.D., Assistant Professor of Internal Medicine and Geriatrics at St. Louis University School of Medicine in St. Louis, Missouri, has studied the short term effects of Preg on memory in humans.

Clinicians

Stan Bazilian, M.D., is a psychiatrist in Philadelphia, Pennsylvania and has used pregnenolone in his practice.

Susan Busse, M.D., is a family practitioner in Palatine, Illinois, who has treated close to 100 individuals with pregnenolone.

Terry Grossman, M.D., in private practice, in Denver, Colorado, has treated about 20 individuals with this hormone. He tells me he has found it to be, in some cases, helpful for osteoarthritis, rheumatoid arthritis, and lupus.

Ascanio Polimeni, M.D., is the director of the Menopause and PMS Center of Milan and Rome.

Dharma Singh Khalsa, M.D., is the Medical Director of the Alzheimer's Prevention Foundation in Tuscon, Arizona, and the author of *Brain Longevity* (Warner, 1997). Dr. Khalsa prescribes pregnenolone and DHEA for age-related memory loss and early Alzheimer's.

Annette Stoesser, M.D., in private practice in Roswell, New Mexico, has taken pregnenolone herself on and off for three years and has treated many patients with it, primarily for memory and energy improvement.

Karlis Ullis, M.D., Assistant Clinical Professor, University of California, Los Angeles, and in private practice, Santa Monica, California, is currently coordinating, with me, clinical studies on pregnenolone.

Paul Yanick, Ph.D., from Montclair, New Jersey, has coordinated, with other physicians, the therapy of over 100 individuals with pregnenolone.

INTRODUCTION

I f you want to achieve optimum health and well-being, you have to learn how to do it yourself. Most doctors don't have the time to teach you everything about the ideal diet, health-promoting lifestyle, suitable mental outlook, proper exercise, and the right supplements. Although doctors may excel at treating a particular medical emergency, most are not experts in health maintenance and have little knowledge about nutritional therapy. Until this changes, you're basically on your own.

One supplement currently available over the counter is pregnenolone, a natural hormone that can, among other things, help improve your mood, memory, and energy level. Unfortunately, few formal studies have been conducted with pregnenolone, and few are likely in the near future. Therefore, much of our current knowledge comes from a limited number of published studies, the experience of physicians, and from anecdotes.

Chances are, your doctor does not know much about pregnenolone, since there have not been any articles discussing its clinical use in the standard medical journals. Does this mean that you should self-medicate with pregnenolone? No. I recommend you consult with your health care practitioner. If he or she is not familiar with this hormone, loan or give them this book.

Doctors are not being adequately exposed to natural therapeutic options because they primarily read medical journals sponsored by pharmaceutical companies. Yet the

---

The Use of Natural Therapies in Medicine

While natural therapies will never replace all pharmaceuticals, they do deserve a place in medicine. Here are a few areas where natural therapies could compete with pharmaceutical drugs:

- Melatonin versus prescription sleeping pills.

- DHEA partially or mostly substituting for synthetic testosterone.

- DHEA partially reducing the need for antidepressants, especially in the elderly.

- Pregnenolone partially reducing the need for antidepressants.

- Soy products lowering the required dosages for estrogen replacement.

- Glucosamine lessening the need for nonsteroidal anti-inflammatory drugs used in osteoarthritis.

- Zinc lozenges replacing many of the cold medicines and the antibiotics that are inappropriately prescribed to fight colds. (Patients often visit a medical office and insist on receiving an antibiotic for a viral upper respiratory infection. Doctors have been known to comply and hand out the unnecessary prescription.)

---

public is learning about natural therapies through books, health magazines, newspapers, and the electronic media. As a consequence, a mini-revolution has started and is gaining momentum; patients are becoming more knowledgeable and self-empowered. They are requesting that their doctors keep up with them. I have little doubt the medical education system will change and improve over the next few years, exposing more doctors to natural treatment options. We are likely to see a wider acceptance of nutrients and hormones in standard medical practice. The pharmaceutical industry will see this as an economic threat—and perhaps there will be a backlash, including the spread of misinformation about the "dangers" of some of these nutrients.

There are many other situations where natural nutritional therapies could replace, or be combined with, existing pharmaceutical drugs. This is a very exciting time for the natural therapy movement. I hope to help it along by providing up-to-date, balanced, and accurate information. *Pregenenolone: Nature's Feel Good Hormone* is a comprehensive, and balanced, evaluation of all aspects of this hormone. I expect this balanced information will counter some of the extreme opinions—excessive hype from promoters, and unreasonable skepticism from critics. The truth lies somewhere between these extremes.

THE AUTHOR'S PERSONAL PREGNENOLONE EXPERIENCE

In March of 1996, I learned that pregnenolone was just starting to be sold over the counter. I already knew that it was a hormone, and that some mice studies had found it to be a potent memory enhancer, but I had no idea what effect it had on humans. I called a number of my colleagues, but none had personally taken this hormone. No one seemed to know what it did. Having a strong sense of curiosity, and a bent towards adventure, I purchased a bottle of 10 milligram (mg) pills.

I should mention that before I write about supplements, I first try them on myself. In addition to experimenting with DHEA, I have done so with melatonin and creatine. Treating patients with these supplements and studying the published research are important, but there's no substitute for a personal trial. Can one be a competent romance novelist never having been passionately in love?

I first tried one pill in the morning and felt no effect. I continued taking 10 mg each morning for the next few days. Nothing. A year earlier, when I was experimenting with DHEA, I had felt an increase in energy the very first day I had

5

taken 10 mg. Thinking to myself that perhaps pregnenolone didn't have a noticeable influence on the human brain, I was about to give it up. Curiosity urged me to continue.

I increased the dosage to 20 mg each morning. I could now barely tell something was going on—perhaps I was a little more alert—but the effect was subtle.

A few days later, I increased the dosage to 30 mg and went about my routine, forgetting that I had taken it. Based on the experience of the previous few days, I didn't expect to feel anything significant. I was considering putting an end to my pregnenolone experiment in order to go on to another hormone or nutrient. However, that evening, while taking a stroll with a friend on the beachfront walk in Venice, California, I could feel something clearly happening. A mellow, steady, persistent feeling of well-being—like a mild euphoria—had imperceptibly come on. Even though I normally feel good, this was different, and better. I became more conscious of my surroundings. Flowers growing in the front gardens of the ocean homes seemed brighter and prettier. I stopped to touch them, and sniffed a yellow-colored rose in full bloom. A mosaic on the door of a beach house caught my eye. Examining it closer, I noticed that it was a scene of tall redwood trees with a curving blue stream running through the middle. My friend graciously accommodated my request that we stare at this mosaic and observe all of its fine details. It dawned on me that I had walked by this house many times before without paying much attention to this artwork. As I continued walking with my friend, my attention focused on the architecture of the homes. I started noticing the patterns of the stones, the shapes of windows, doorways, and porticos, and other details. The palm trees lining the walk appeared Caribbean island-like picturesque. Everything seemed more beautiful and intriguing. I felt a sense of childish wonder, that "everything was okay." How special and enchanting life could be!

I didn't take any pregnenolone the next day, yet my sense of well-being continued, but on a more subtle level. During a midday break, as I sat on my office chair lost in my thoughts, staring out through the balcony at the slow, undulating waves melting into the jetty rocks, I reflected about the previous evening's delightful experience. A number of thoughts, ideas, and possibilities raced through my brain. Pregnenolone was so interesting—and so unknown. I wondered what kind of response this non-prescription, perception-enhancing hormone would receive from the public, the medical establishment, the government, and the media. Would it be accepted or scorned? I also considered all the potential uses of this hormone in the fields of psychiatry and medicine, and how it could be helpful in restoring youthful awareness to older individuals whose production of this hormone has declined with the decades.

Learning more about pregnenolone became my passion. I started recommending it to patients and friends who were willing to give it a try. I talked to everyone I knew who might have used this hormone. Over the next few months, I contacted many more colleagues. Only a few had used pregnenolone in their practices, and in most cases their experience was limited. I then did a complete and thorough review of the scientific literature, looking at long-buried studies dating back to the 1940s.

Since my first days of experimentation, I have tried a number of pregnenolone products and a variety of forms, including pills, capsules, micronized capsules, sublingual tablets, and skin creams. There are often subtle, and not so subtle, distinctions among different forms, and different brands. I've also tried a variety of dosages. Initially, it took me a few days, and 30 mg, to feel the effects of pregnenolone, but now I can notice the effects even on as low a dosage as 5 mg—and sometimes within an hour of dosing. I have taken pregnenolone at home, in the office, on sunny days, cloudy days, while walking in the mist, in heavy downpours, on the beach, hiking in the mountains, listening to music, at parties, eating out, traveling in Italy, meandering through a shopping mall, and in a variety of other settings. Furthermore, I have interviewed prominent researchers in the field, and I continue to evaluate the latest published research. I and a colleague, Dr. Karlis Ullis, are doing clinical evaluations of many patients on this hormone. In addition, I am cooperating with the Southwest College of Naturopathic Medicine in Tempe, Arizona, on a study evaluating the role of pregnenolone and premenstrual syndrome. In the following chapters, you will find detailed information never before published.

I'm 39 years old, and therefore too young to take pregnenolone regularly. But I am currently taking this hormone about once a week, in the range of 5 to 20 mg. I plan to do so until my late forties or fifties, when I'll begin using it more frequently. Hopefully, by then, we'll have a much better understanding of this once-forgotten, yet fascinating, hormone.

In the next chapter, I'll explain what Preg is and how its potential benefits were ignored for so long.

CHAPTER 2

THE GRANDMOTHER OF ALL STEROID HORMONES

Provides a peaceful, harmonious, euphoric well-being
Enhances alertness and awareness
Heightens visual and auditory perception
Reduces stress
Improves memory and clarity of thinking
Makes you feel younger, more vibrant, and happier

P regnenolone, if used appropriately, can improve the quality of your life.

What is Pregnenolone?

Pregnenolone, Preg for short, is a *hormone* made primarily in the adrenal glands (see the diagram on page 10), but also in the brain, liver, skin, testicles, and ovaries. Please note that all words in italics are defined in the glossary.

The chemical name for Preg is 3-alpha-hydroxy-5-beta-pregnen-20-one. When you swallow a Preg pill, it makes its way into the bloodstream and then travels around to the rest of the body. It then enters a variety of tissues and cells, where

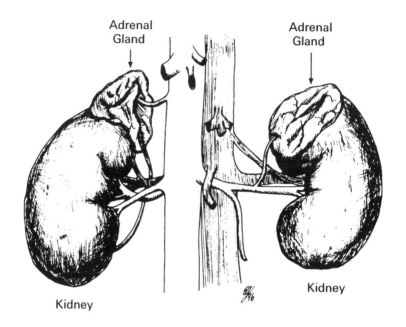

it is used as Preg or is converted into DHEA, which in turn has the ability to be converted into *androgens, estrogens,* and other steroids (see page 18).

There's another pathway that Preg can take. It can be *metabolized* into progesterone. This is what makes Preg different from DHEA. It has the ability to form other hormones such as progesterone. DHEA has often been called the "Mother Hormone." Preg is the mother of DHEA and progesterone, and I call it "The Grandmother of All Steroid Hormones."

Historical background

Preg was first prepared in a laboratory in 1934. Many human studies done in the 1940s showed that Preg could combat fatigue, ease arthritic aches and pains, improve well-being, fight stress, and enhance thinking ability (Hoagland; 1944, Pincus, 1944, 1945).

In 1950, a full review article was published in the *Journal of Clinical Endocrinology* by Dr. Edward Henderson and colleagues from the division of Clinical Research at Schering Corporation in Bloomfield, New Jersey. Their article begins quite auspiciously:

> *Publications on the use of adrenocortical hormones in the treatment of rheumatoid arthritis and other collagen diseases have stimulated further research to determine the activity of steroids that have heretofore received little attention. Among those now being studied, pregnenolone appears to have certain advantages that should mark this compound as worthy of careful inquiry. It has an extremely low order of toxicity, has not shown any adverse effect on endocrine physiology, and has shown some promise in the treatment of rheumatoid arthritis.*

Shortly thereafter the research on Preg abruptly stopped. Why?

Natural hormones just don't get no respect

In the late 1940s—about the same time the Preg studies were being conducted—cortisone, another closely related hormone, was being evaluated. When cortisone was given to individuals with rheumatoid arthritis, there were outstanding short-term improvements. Photographs of these remarkable recoveries were circulated, and the medical community was impressed. Cortisone trumped Preg and stole the limelight. Scientists basically put Preg aside to focus on cortisone. The structure of cortisone was altered to make similar molecules such as dexamethasone and prednisone, much more powerful steroids. Dexamethasone and other similar corticosteroids could be patented, so a pharmaceutical company could make a lot of money on them. It was only years later that medicine discovered some of the dangers of long-term high-dose corticosteroid use, including immune system depression.

Since the 1950s, Preg has virtually gone into obscurity with only rare mentions in the medical literature. A review of Medline, the computer system that records all articles published in scientific journals, shows only a few studies published on Preg in 1996 and 1997, with only a couple involving human subjects. Enormous amounts of research have been conducted on the metabolites, or byproducts, of Preg, including progesterone, *aldosterone*, and *cortisol* (especially synthetic corticosteroids). DHEA has been the subject of a fair share of research, though less so than the metabolites of DHEA, such as estrogens and androgens.

John Morley, M.D., a steroid hormone researcher from the University of St. Louis in Missouri, says, "I think Preg has potentially extremely exciting properties. Drug companies have zero interest in Preg since it can't be patented and they can't make a profit from it."

Is Preg safe?

As I learn more about melatonin, Preg, and DHEA from using them myself, treating patients, discussing the effects with thousands of users, exchanging notes with other physicians, reading letters sent to our research center, and reviewing the latest published studies, I am becoming more and more convinced that we should be treating these hormones with utmost respect. Hormones have broad, and significant, effects on a variety of cells, tissues, and organs. Even small amounts can notably alter countless chemical reactions within our bodies. Proper usage of hormones can be very beneficial, leading to dramatic improvements in health and quality of life. But carelessly swallowing high dosages will be counterproductive, leading to unfavorable long-term consequences—perhaps even shortening life span.

In short-term rodent and human studies done thus far, Preg appears to be safe, with no apparent toxicity noted.

Rodent studies—When mice were given 5,000 mg of Preg per kilogram (kg) of body weight, no acute toxicity was produced and there were no deaths (Henderson, 1950). One kilogram is 2.2 pounds, so this would be equivalent, by weight ratio, to giving a 70 kg (154 pound) human 350,000 mg. Most of the pills sold over the counter are less than 50 mg.

In a long-term study, mice were given 1,000 mg of Preg per kg of body weight three times a week for 50 doses, with no toxic reactions. No changes were noted in red blood cells, white blood cells, hemoglobin, or the weight of body organs. Also, no changes were found in food intake, growth rate, fertility, or the size and condition of offspring (Henderson, 1950).

Human studies—When 25 men were given between 25 and 75 mg of Preg daily, one person developed a rash, which stopped after the Preg was discontinued. None of the other users developed side effects (Tyler, 1943).

In another study, no adverse effects were noted when eight patients received 100 mg of Preg daily by intramuscular injection for 75 days (Henderson, 1950).

McGavack and colleagues, in an article published in 1951, reported using Preg in 59 patients in dosages ranging from 50 to 600 mg intramuscularly from four to 167 days. They wrote, "No toxic reactions to Preg were encountered. Occasional redness, pain and swelling occurred at the site of an injection."

Dr. Gregory Pincus and Dr. Hudson Hoagland were even more confident about Preg's safety. Back in 1944 they wrote:

We should like to point out that we have encountered no deleterious result in connection with the ingestion of pregnenolone in our studies involving several hundred men and women who have taken the medication, in some instances in doses of 100 mg per day, for as long as four months. The substance [Preg] is nontoxic.

For the most part, persons report no subjective experiences after its ingestion, although a considerable number have insisted that they experience a general feeling of well-being and that they tire less easily when taking it.

Dr. Roberts reports that 525 mg of Preg given daily to patients with Alzheimer's disease for three months did not induce any apparent toxicity (personal communication).

The safety of Preg when used regularly for long periods, such as years or decades, has not been formally evaluated. The longest user of Preg I know is Annette, from Roswell, New Mexico. She tells me, "Three years ago I went almost a year taking 200 mg of Preg daily just to see what it would do. Then I cut back the dose and have been taking 50 mg off and on. I haven't noticed any side effects. I play tennis and have less soreness if I'm taking Preg."

Just because researchers have not found any significant side effects with a particular medicine does not mean that it is harmless. Sometimes researchers fail to note obvious reactions. A classic example is the influence of melatonin on dreams. It's hard to believe that none of the published articles on melatonin in scientific journals had ever mentioned that this hormone induced vivid dreaming. I discovered this effect the very first night that I took it. I was the first to publish my observations in *Melatonin: Nature's Sleeping Pill.* How could researchers over a three decade period of melatonin investigation have missed such an obvious finding that I noticed immediately?

The very same thing could happen with Preg. We may find both positive and negative effects that have not been previously discussed in the limited published studies. Please read the precautions in Chapter 11 before starting Preg.

How are Preg supplements manufactured?

There is a plant called wild yam (*Dioscorea* species) that is grown in many parts of the world, especially in Mexico. A pharmaceutical researcher, Dr. Michael Bennett from San Diego, has studied the manufacturing process of steroid compounds extensively and has visited various laboratories. He explains, "Dioscorea contains a compound called *diosgenin* that is the chemical precursor to steroid hormones. In a laboratory, diosgenin is converted into Preg through a series of several chemical processes. The diosgenin content of the Mexican wild yam is the highest in the world. China is another large supplier of diosgenin."

The human body does not have the required enzymes to convert diosgenin into Preg. Therefore, if you swallow pills that are extracts of wild yams, or spread yam creams on your body, you will not get Preg or DHEA. The conversion of diosgenin to Preg must be done in a laboratory. If you want Preg or DHEA, the bottles you buy should state that they contain actual Preg or DHEA, not unprocessed extracts of wild yams. The creams must say they contain actual Preg or DHEA.

Researchers at the University of Arizona School of Medicine in Tucson gave volunteers aged 65 to 82 Dioscorea extracts for three weeks and then DHEA for another three weeks (Araghiniknam, 1996). They found that Dioscorea had no effect on blood DHEA levels, while 85 mg a day of DHEA doubled blood DHEA levels. Interestingly, both treatments reduced blood *triglycerides*, increased HDL *cholesterol* levels, and reduced serum lipid oxidation. This means there's less fat in the blood, and the blood fat that does exist is less likely to create blockages. Both Dioscorea and DHEA were found to have *antioxidant* properties.

Before you run to the health food store and buy yam extracts, please realize that a variety of fresh fruits, vegetables, whole grains, and legumes contain antioxidants. Whether extracts from wild yams offer benefits superior to these healthy foods remains to be seen.

How is Preg made in the body?

The parts of the cell where Preg is made are called mitochondria. These are tiny little enclosures within cells that digest and break down sugars, fats, and proteins. Mitochondria are the chemical factories of a cell, and also are the places where steroids are produced.

The amount of Preg made depends on how much cholesterol is brought to the mitochondria. Cholesterol usually floats within the cell in tiny clumps. When the body needs Preg and other steroids, it brings the cholesterol to the mitochondria, which then break a few chemical bonds from the cholesterol to turn it into Preg (Stocco, 1992).

What other hormones does Preg turn into?

When you take Preg, your body will decide which pathway it will take (see the diagram on page 18). Will it go the DHEA way, or the progesterone direction?

Hans Selye, the well-known pioneer researcher on stress, was first to point out Preg's ability to be converted into different steroids. Back in 1943, he wrote:

> *Pregnenolone distinguishes itself from other steroids because it possesses so many different activities. Thus the compound possesses, at least in traces, every independent main pharmacological action which*

has hitherto been shown to be exhibited by any steroid hormone. In the light of these observations it was tempting to speculate on the possible role of the compound as a hormone-precursor from which the organism may, according to its needs, produce compounds in which one effect is particularly developed at the expense of other activities of the parent substance.

At least 150 steroid hormones are made from Preg. Preg can be converted into DHEA and progesterone, but we're not certain what proportion of ingested Preg is eventually converted into hormones further down the metabolic pathway, such as androgens, estrogens, cortisol, or aldosterone. Also, we often look at a diagram with simple lines going from one hormone to another and think we can predict the action of a hormone in the body based on what it's supposed to be converted into as drawn. It doesn't necessarily work that way in the body. There could be a variety of interconversions between different hormones. As Dr. Morley told me, "The hormonal system can be driven backward and forward; it's not just a straight path from one metabolite to another. The system is a lot more complicated than we think. There are a lot of interconversions that we don't know of."

Why take Preg instead of DHEA?

Let's keep in mind that Preg has actions independent of its conversion into other hormones. Many of the effects of Preg could be due to its own actions, and not due to its conversion into DHEA or progesterone. Furthermore, Preg's concentration in the brain is several times that of DHEA (Baulieu, 1996).

James F. Flood, Ph.D., of the Medical Research Service at the St. Louis University School of Medicine, is one of the world's foremost researchers on Preg, especially its influence

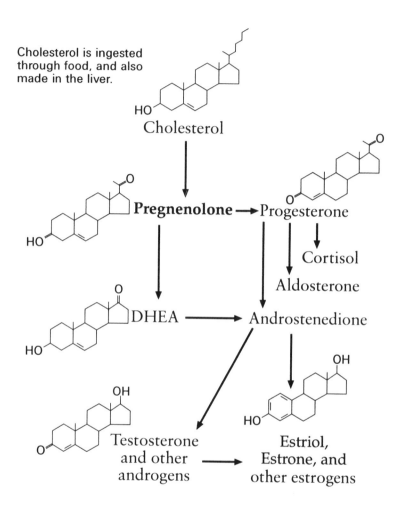

Cholesterol is ingested through food, and also made in the liver.

Cholesterol

Pregnenolone → Progesterone

Cortisol

Aldosterone

DHEA ——→ Androstenedione

Testosterone and other androgens

Estriol, Estrone, and other estrogens

Please note that some metabolic steps have been skipped in order to simplify this diagram

Metabolism of Cholesterol to Pregnenolone and Other Hormones

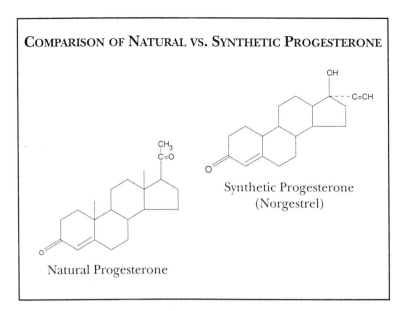

COMPARISON OF NATURAL VS. SYNTHETIC PROGESTERONE

Synthetic Progesterone
(Norgestrel)

Natural Progesterone

Dr. John Lee believes that "In Western industrialized culture, pharmaceutical companies buy natural progesterone (derived from yams) and then chemically alter its molecular form to produce the various progestins, which, being not found in nature, are patentable and therefore more profitable. Most physicians are unaware their prescription progestins are made from progesterone (from yams)."[16]

One drawback of progestogen is that its chemical structure is different from the progesterone in your body. Progestogen also doesn't act like your own progesterone does. It can't convert into other steroid hormones. When choosing a hormone treatment, it is important to remember that progesterone is the primary building block for all other steroid hormones and this alone distinguishes natural progesterone from progestogen. Instead of binding to the progesterone receptors in your body, most of progestogen binds to androgen (male hormone) receptors. This means progestogen has mild male-inducing effects like increased facial hair. There are minimal, if any, side effects with natural progesterone.

on memory. He tells me, "A major difference between Preg and DHEA is that Preg is comparatively found in higher amounts in the central nervous system but not as much in peripheral tissues, while DHEA is found in higher amounts in peripheral tissues but in lower amounts in the central nervous system. Preg has an effect on the central nervous system in much lower doses than other steroid hormones. It probably affects different regions of the brain compared to DHEA."

One advantage that Preg has over DHEA is that it is less androgenic or virilizing. That is, individuals who easily get pimples or facial hair from DHEA would be less likely to do so on Preg. (A 10 mg dose of DHEA can sometimes induce a small pimple on my face while it takes 40 or more mg of Preg to do the same.) And Preg seems to have a more potent anti-inflammatory capability. Both hormones, though, seem to be similar in producing feelings of well-being. I would venture that DHEA has more libido-enhancing influences than Preg.

There are many circumstances, such as hormone replacement therapy in older individuals, where it may be advantageous to take both hormones. We'll discuss this issue in Chapter 4.

How much Preg is made daily?

There's too little research on Preg to know for certain the exact production in humans. However, a small study conducted in 1967 by Dr. Wang and colleagues in London gives us an approximation.

When Preg circulates in the bloodstream, it does so attached to oxygen and a mineral called sulfur. This combination of one sulfur and four oxygen atoms is known as sulfate (SO_4). The sulfate attached to Preg makes it more water soluble, and thus easier to circulate and transport in the bloodstream. Preg sulfate is denoted as Preg-S. Wang and colleagues estimate that the blood level of Preg sulfate in adult men is about 10 micrograms per 100 milliliters, and that the average human production would be about 14 mg per day. Of course, this is a very rough estimate. The amount would be less in the elderly and in many cases there would be significant variation between individuals.

Do Preg levels stay constant throughout life?

The production of many of our hormones declines with age. This is true of melatonin, DHEA, and Preg. For instance, it is estimated that our bodies make 60 percent less Preg at age 75 than at age 35 (Roberts, 1995). Again, this is a rough estimate, since few studies have formally evaluated Preg levels through-out life. Dr. Morley tells me, "The data we have reviewed shows Preg levels decline with age in a manner similar to that of DHEA."

The decrease in Preg production can lead to the decline in other hormones that are synthesized from it, including DHEA, progesterone, and dozens of other intermediary steroid hormones.

Can I be tested for Preg levels in my body?

Yes, it is possible to test for Preg levels in your blood. We'll discuss the advantages and shortcomings of testing in Chapter 10.

How is the production of Preg monitored?

Hormones released from the pituitary gland regulate the amount of Preg that is made. The pituitary gland is called the "master" gland since it is involved in coordinating the many hormones in our bodies.

Three of the regulating hormones released by the pituitary gland are leutenizing hormone, follicle-stimulating hormone, and *ACTH*. There's always interaction and communication between the pituitary gland located in the brain and the rest of the organs in our body. When the production of hormones by the adrenal glands is too high, the pituitary gland sends signals to reduce production. When the amount of certain adrenal hormones is too low, the pituitary gland again sends signals, this time to stimulate further production. There's always a balance to be maintained. This balance is called homeostasis.

There are enzymes in cells that convert cholesterol to Preg, and it is made in varying amounts in different parts of our bodies.

Will taking Preg stop my own body's production?

We don't know the full answer to this question, but we do know that ingesting low amounts of DHEA does not lead to a feedback inhibition. I suspect low doses of Preg will not stop our body's natural production, but more research is needed.

As we'll discover in the next chapter, The Grandmother of All Steroid Hormones has an enormous influence on well-being. It is the ultimate Feel Good Hormone. Preg can have a positive influence, either by itself, or likely in combination with other nutrients, hormones, medicines, and therapies, in improving the health and quality of life for much of the population. After all, isn't it preferable to go through life feeling good?

CHAPTER 3

YOUR BRAIN ON PREG

The use of hormones such as Preg to specifically improve mental function has generally been overlooked by the medical profession. The primary focus of hormone supplementation, such as estrogen replacement therapy, has been on strictly physical benefits, such as the prevention of osteoporosis and the improvement of cardiovascular health. Recently, however, doctors have realized that estrogen replacement in women can positively influence brain function, including reducing the risk of Alzheimer's disease (see Chapter 4 for information on hormone replacement therapy and Chapter 7 for information on Alzheimer's disease). In this chapter, I wish to propose and discuss the concept that Preg and DHEA play a significant role in brain health.

Your brain makes Preg

Until 1981, scientists thought that steroids found in the brain came from elsewhere in the body. We now know that the brain has the capacity to use cholesterol to produce Preg and other steroids (Warner, 1995). Our brains and neural systems contain large amounts of steroid *precursors*, such as cholesterol, and also contain the necessary enzymes to convert cholesterol into a variety of steroid hormones, including Preg (Majewska, 1989). In fact, levels of Preg are many times higher in the human brain and neural tissues than they are in the bloodstream (Lanthier, 1986; Robel, 1995). Steroids made in the brain are called neurosteroids. Scientists still haven't discovered all the steroids that our bodies and brains make. At last count, over 150 steroid hormones had been identified.

Medicine has not made an active effort in treating "normal" declines in mental functioning. When an older patient goes to his or her physician and complains, "Doctor, I can't seem to think as clearly or remember things as well as I used to," the response often is, "Well, what do you expect? That's just part of the aging process."

Fortunately, many doctors are realizing that there are now several options to help older individuals maintain optimum brain function. The brain needs to be exercised. This can be done by maintaining a career or part-time employment, by getting involved in hobbies or artistic endeavors, or by taking adult education classes. Solving crossword puzzles, watching *Jeopardy*, and engaging in physical exercise will also help. Supplementation with various vitamins, nutrients, herbs, hormones, and pharmaceutical agents can be extremely beneficial. I believe Preg, DHEA, and other hormones can play a crucial role in improving or maintaining mental capacity. In addition to memory enhancement, these hormones play a role in returning some of the alertness and enchantment with life normally felt in our youth that so gradually diminishes over the decades.

Wouldn't it make more sense to spend more research money evaluating the effects of DHEA, Preg, and other hormones on mood, intelligence, and memory in middle aged and older individuals?

Preg influences brain chemistry

I am 100 percent convinced that taking Preg leads to changes in awareness and alertness. I vouch from my personal experience. But what exactly does Preg do in the brain?

Scientists are still in the process of discovering the variety of ways steroid hormones influence brain chemistry. Research in this area is still in its infancy. However, I will discuss what we know thus far.

There are many *receptors* on our brain cells that respond to a variety of brain chemicals. For instance, endorphins, chemicals that can reduce pain, have their own receptors on certain brain cells. So does *serotonin*. GABA is the brain chemical that is the principal inhibitory *neurotransmitter* in the brain. Stimulation of GABA receptors leads to mental slowing, relaxation, and slumber. Sedatives, such as Valium, calm us by attaching on GABA receptors and stimulating them. When a drug or hormone stimulates a receptor, it is called an agonist. When it prevents a receptor from working, it is called an antagonist.

Valium is called a GABA agonist. Preg, though, has mixed functions, both stimulating GABA receptors in some parts of the brain while inhibiting others (Robel, 1995).

The retinas in our eyes are even known to make Preg (Guarneri, 1995). When I take Preg, I notice an improved visual clarity; this can happen within an hour of dosing. Could this effect be due to the influence on GABA receptors processes in the cells of the retina?

Valium and Preg are not the only drugs or hormones that act on GABA receptors. Various medicines such as anticonvulsants (Dilantin), anesthetics, and other medicines do so, too.

It is likely that Preg interacts with many other receptors in the brain. The human brain is a very difficult organ to study. Researchers are constantly learning more of its secrets. It may surprise you to learn that our brains contain an enormous numbers of brain cells—at least 100 billion neurons! In addition, there are 900 billion other brain cells that support and nourish these neurons. The full count is one trillion— one million times one million. The number of brain cells decreases with age. The amount of Preg and other steroids produced in the brain also lessen with age. This decline in steroids prevents us from functioning at our best. We are not able to think as clearly, our memory falters—and we forget where we put our car keys. Our ability to be creative and make rapid calculations decreases. These are all symptoms of old age. Is it possible that by supplying ourselves with supplements of Preg and other hormones, we can reverse or slow down some of these declines in mental function?

We don't have all the answers yet but, in the future, the therapeutic potential for Preg and DHEA could include various neurological conditions, some forms of dementia, and especially the gradual mental deterioration that occurs in almost everyone as the decades relentlessly march on.

Memory and thinking

Preg is known to stimulate the *NMDA* receptors in the brain (Wu, 1991). These receptors play an important role in regulating the function and form of synapses, or points of contact, between our neurons, and thus influence learning and memory. Aging is thought to be associated with a decline in the number of NMDA receptors, which may partly account for loss of learning ability and memory. Interestingly, the administration of acetyl-l-carnitine (a nutrient and antioxidant found in stores) slows the age-associated reduction in the number of NMDA receptors in rodents (Castorina, 1993).

Dr. Flood tells me that Preg also has a profound influence on the acetylcholine system. *Acetylcholine* is a brain chemical intimately involved in memory. In fact, abnormalities with the acetylcholine system are a major problem in Alzheimer's disease.

Thorough studies involving Preg and memory in humans have not yet been published. However, much research has been done with mice (Isaacson, 1995; Flood, 1992, 1995a). When as few as 150 *molecules* of Preg are injected into certain parts of the mouse brain, there is a significant enhancement of memory. Dr. Flood wrote in his 1992 article, "Pregnenolone and pregnenolone sulfate, for which receptors have not yet been demonstrated, may exert their effects by serving as precursors for the formation of a panoply of different steroids, ensuring near-optimal modulation of transcription of immediate-early genes required for achieving the plastic changes of memory processes." A few years later, in 1995, Drs. Flood, Morley, and Roberts concluded, "Preg is the most potent memory enhancer yet reported." In another article published in *Physiology and Behavior* in 1995, Dr. Flood adds, "Preg, DHEA and testosterone decrease with age. This decrease may contribute to the age-related deficit in learning and memory."

Drs. Baulieu and Robel are just as convinced about Preg's effect on memory. In a 1996 article published in the *Journal of Endocrinology*, they state:

> We evaluated the cognitive performances of aged rats. Some aged rats are impaired, whereas others perform as well as young ones. Memory performances of 29 aged rats (about 24 months old) were measured in a water maze and in a two-trial recognition task. At the completion of the behavioral study, animals were sacrificed and their brain was removed for analysis of Preg-S concentrations in selected areas. A striking observation was the significant positive correlation between the concentration of Preg-S in the hippocampus and memory performance. Namely, animals with better performances had greater levels of Preg-S.

These results support the possible neuroprotective role of Preg-S (and likewise DHEAS) against neurodegenerative processes.

In 1996, Drs. Melchior and Ritzmann at the Department of Psychiatry, Olive View branch of UCLA in Sylmar, California, gave 0.5 gm/kg of alcohol to mice and found that this impaired their memory. When they gave low doses of Preg or DHEA, they found that these neurosteroids were capable of blocking the memory-impairing effect of the ethanol. They say, "The influence of these compounds on memory and their interactions on this behavior are consistent with their actions on the GABA system." This raises the question whether Preg could be beneficial for those who have memory impairment due to prior years of alcohol or drug overuse.

A human memory study

Rahmawati Sih, M.D., Assistant Professor of Internal Medicine and Geriatrics at St. Louis University School of Medicine at St. Louis, Missouri, became interested in Preg while working with Dr. Morley on the effects of this hormone in rodents. In 1996, she conducted a brief study in which she administered a one-time dose of 10 to 500 mg of Preg to humans to test the immediate effects on memory. The results have not been fully analyzed and statistically correlated, but preliminary evidence shows that the higher the Preg dosage, the better the memory performance. No side effects were reported in this study. Dr. Sih tells me that a few volunteers noticed a decrease in their arthritis symptoms as well.

I believe taking high doses of Preg can be detrimental. Perhaps low amounts, such as 5 to 15 mg, could enhance memory just as well when given for prolonged periods. Dr. Flood agrees: "Preg could be helpful in improving memory, but taking too much will be counterproductive, impairing cognitive function."

Dr. Sih is currently giving Preg to older individuals through a grant provided by the American Federation of Aging Research. She is testing the effect of Preg on such physical and psychological parameters as strength, gait, mood, sexual drive, and energy.

Dharma Singh Khalsa, M.D., author of *Brain Longevity*, says, "A common thing my older patients, especially women, tell me, is that during a conversation Preg helps them find the word they're looking for."

Other natural nutrients and herbs to consider for memory improvement include ginkgo biloba, phosphotidylserine, B-complex vitamins, and acetyl-l-carnitine.

Preg and mood

In addition to a decline in memory, some middle-aged and many older individuals also have a decline in their mood. Seniors often do not notice that they are not as happy and excited about life as they once were. If mood drops even lower, we call this "depression," and doctors will attempt to treat it with pharmaceutical antidepressants. These antidepressants may often help, but they will not address the primary problem if the low mood is a result of a deficiency of brain steroid hormones. I believe that Preg will eventually be found to have a role in treating depression and will be used either by itself, or in combination with hormones, vitamins, and nutrients. If this initial therapy fails, then Preg can be tried in combination with lower doses of herbs (such as St. John's wort) or pharmaceutical antidepressants. Of course, before treating depression with supplements and drugs, doctors will need to rule out any medical condition that could be causing it.

A milder form of depression, which is estimated to

affect 5 to 10 percent of the population, is dysthymia. Symptoms include feelings of helplessness, fatigue, low self-esteem, over- or undereating, sleep irregularity, and poor motivation. It is usually diagnosed in females between the ages of 15 and 55. Individuals often live for years with this disorder and blame themselves for their low moods. The current accepted therapy for dysthymia is the use of tricyclic antidepressants, such as imipramine and desipramine, as well as some of the newer serotonin re-uptake inhibitors, including fluoxetine and sertraline. Could the temporary use of Preg, as a mood-improving boost, help sufferers get back on track?

Karlis Ullis, M.D., a physician in private practice in Santa Monica, California, is collaborating with me in evaluating the clinical effects of Preg, specifically its influence on mood. Dr. Ullis has tried Preg himself. He tells me, "Preg provides a constant, stable, all day long, smooth and even well-being. I notice the effects within an hour or two of taking 10 mg. I'm also more focused dur-ing the day when I'm seeing patients. Based on prelimi-nary evidence, I believe Preg has a role to play as an anti-depressant."

We have indirect evidence that Preg is involved in mood disorders. Researchers sampled Preg and proges-terone levels in the cerebrospinal fluid (CSF) of 27 patients suffering from depression and in that of 10 healthy volun-teers (George, 1994). CSF circulates throughout the spinal column and brain, thus reflecting any major changes in brain chemistry. The results were intriguing: depressed patients had lower levels of Preg in their CSF than did the healthy volunteers. Progesterone levels were the same in both patients and volunteers. The researchers state, "CSF pregnenolone is decreased in subjects with affective ill-ness, particularly during episodes of active depression.

Further research into the role of neuroactive steroids in mood regulation is warranted." For dosage information regarding Preg and mood elevation, see Chapter 9.

Organic Psychopharmacology?

If future studies show that long-term use of DHEA and Preg have no significant side effects, I believe that these hormones will create a revolution in our current under-standing of and therapy for depression, especially in middle-aged and older individuals.

I have personally talked to hundreds of Preg users. I'm consistently told by them that Preg improves their sense of well-being. However, in some cases, the effects are subtle and not everyone notices them.

Many doctors may find that Preg's mood-elevating effects would reduce the need for antidepressant drugs. If a patient is already on these antidepressant drugs, a physician can attempt to lower the doses, and perhaps the medicines can, in some cases, eventually be stopped. We know that serotonin re-uptake inhibitors often have unpleasant side effects such as nausea and loss of libido. The last thing a depressed patient wants is to lose his or her sex drive. Loss of sexual drive leads to the loss of an important form of nurturing, physical intimacy.

We may also find that, in some people, Preg and DHEA in combination would be more effective. Receptors for these hormones are already there on our DNA. We could call this new, natural brain therapy "Organic Psychopharmacology."

The following are some other areas where I feel Preg should be studied.

The age of anxiety

We all know individuals who suffer from excessive worry, irritability, and tension. They may have bodily symptoms, including increased heart rate and high blood pressure; gastrointestinal symptoms, such as bloating and ulcer-type stomach pains; and a variety of neurologic symptoms, including headaches and dizziness. Most doctors treat anxiety by prescribing *benzodiazepines* such as diazepam (Valium), alprazolam, and others. Since Preg provides a steadiness of mood and a sense of harmonious balance, it could theoretically be helpful.

In one study on mice, Preg-S caused an increase in anxiety-type behavior at higher doses (10 and 1 microgram/kg), but reduced anxiety-type behavior in a lower dose (0.1 microgram/kg) (Melchior, 1994). It's possible the same could occur in humans.

Other anxiety disorders include panic attacks and OBD (obsessive-compulsive disorder). It would be interesting to find out whether low doses of Preg can play a role in ameliorating these conditions—maybe even in treating phobias.

Chronic pain disorders

There are case histories of patients with chronic complaints of pain who visit doctor after doctor, yet in whom no medical cause for the pain can be found. Often their symptoms far exceed the medical findings and no therapy or medicine seems to work. Some of these patients could be suffering from anxiety, depression, or just a lack of excitement about life. Since Preg can induce good mood, energy, and feelings of well-being, it could offer a novel therapeutic approach for these patients.

Creativity

The clear thinking and vision, enhanced alertness, focused-concentration, improved memory, and, in general, overall better mental function on Preg can be occasionally taken advantage of by artists, writers, and actors. Artists would appreciate the visual enhancement, which leads to a clearer perception of colors and patterns. At times, perhaps, Preg can even be helpful to scientists, mathematicians, and inventors.

Manic-depression

Also known as bipolar disorder, symptoms start in late teens and early adult life. During the manic phase, there is elation with hyperactivity, increased irritability, and little need for sleep. The over-enthusiastic quality of the mood and the expansive behavior initially attract others, but the irritability, mood swings, aggressive behavior, and grandiosity usually lead to marked interpersonal difficulties (*Current Medical Diagnosis*, 1997).

Since Preg provides a balanced and harmonious disposition, it would be interesting to explore the use of this hormone in low doses in the manic and depressive stages of this condition.

An especially good area to investigate Preg's therapeutic potential is in those who have a cyclothymic disorder. This refers to a milder form of manic-depression, in which there are lower highs and higher lows.

Personality disorders

As a physician, I have seen, talked with, and examined thousands of patients over the years. I have noticed that a lot of people who have difficult personalities or maladaptive behaviors are often suffering from low self-esteem, lack of self-confidence, or low mood, or are possibly experiencing high levels of stress. By elevating mood and reducing stress, Preg might offer some help and allow such individuals to deal more constructively with everyday problems.

Sex drive

Anecdotal experience tells us that Preg does not seem to have much of an influence on libido. DHEA, though, being metabolically closer to testosterone, does enhance sex drive in the majority of users.

In the next chapter, we will look at how Preg can be used as part of a replacement therapy program.

CHAPTER 4

PREGNENOLONE REPLACEMENT THERAPY (PRT)

Rage, rage against the dying of the light!

I recalled this powerful line from Dylan Thomas' moving poem, "Do not go gentle into that good night" as I read a letter sent to me by Robert, a gentleman from Perth, Scotland. Robert writes:

> *At the age of 66 I'm on a senescent decline. I had a cardiac operation which left residual problems. My main interest now lies in the area of delaying this onslaught, and after spending a year experimenting with various substances, my focus has narrowed to hormonal supplementation. My daily regimen now consists of:*
>
> > *DHEA —10 mg*
> >
> > *Pregnenolone —10 mg*
> >
> > *Melatonin—0.5 mg (most nights)*
>
> *The cumulative effect of the past 12 months' experience is that I am more contented, feel healthier, fitter,*

energized, and in these days of maturation, I frequently experience that previously seldom-found feel good factor. These hormones have put me back on the saddle again. Indeed, on many days I now feel happy. It's been a long time since I've been able to admit to that kind of feeling.

I subscribe to the view about not wishing to wait for 20 or 30 years for conclusive evidence to accumulate—I just don't have that time scale available. And as I'm already on my way out, I'm more than happy to risk going . . . my way!

In this chapter, we'll see how pregnenolone replacement therapy (PRT) can be used to help improve quality of life.

Reversing the downward slope?

During routine hormone replacement therapy for post-menopausal women, doctors prescribe mainly estrogen (and sometimes progesterone or a synthetic progestin). Recently, doctors have also been recommending that older men receive replacement *testosterone*. Research is accumulating, though, that suggests replacing other hormones that diminish with age is also appropriate—not only for women, but for men, too. Therefore, in this chapter, when I refer to "hormone replacement therapy," I will be discussing a variety of hormones in addition to estrogen, progesterone, and testosterone.

Not all the hormones in our bodies decline with age. Levels of cortisol, made by the adrenal glands, and *insulin*, made by the pancreas, stay relatively the same or even increase. Thyroid hormone levels vary. But levels of Preg, DHEA, melatonin, growth hormone, progesterone, estrogens, and testosterone all decrease with age.

The decline in the production of hormones due to

aging, or as a consequence of illness or chronic stress, can have a profoundly negative influence on a number of body tissues. All these hormones have the ability to enter most cells of the body, go to the DNA, induce the formations of a variety of enzymes and proteins, and significantly influence the function of cells and tissues.

Let's look at the roles played by the following hormones in hormone replacement therapy:

• **Estrogen**—This is the main female hormone, and the one that is usually given to postmenopausal women. Keep in mind that men's bodies also make estrogen.

• **Progesterone**—This is a natural version of synthetic progestins. Currently, it is added to estrogen in therapy for postmenopausal women who have intact uteruses.

• **Testosterone**—This is the main male hormone, although women's bodies make it, too.

• **DHEA**—This hormone is the mother for the sex hormones, including estrogens and testosterone (see the diagram on page 18).

• **Preg**—This is the mother of DHEA, and the grandmother of all the adrenal steroid hormones, including the sex hormones.

When discussing hormone replacement therapy, it is simplistic to discuss Preg by itself because all of these hormones are closely tied together. Thus, in this chapter, I'll discuss the benefits of combination therapy.

DHEA, which is converted into androgens and estrogens, can induce health benefits. Perhaps by giving Preg, or by using a combination of Preg and DHEA, we could achieve an even more harmonious balance. Dr. Eugene Roberts, in his 1995 review article, writes:

Restoration of normal steroid patterns by adminis-
tration of Preg alone or together with much smaller than
currently employed amounts of other steroids is likely to
be less physiologically disturbing than is administration
of arbitrarily selected amounts of more potent substances
that derive from it, e.g., cortisone, sex steroids, or aldos-
terone, because myriad feedback inhibitory foci exist in
steroid formation beginning with the synthesis of Preg
from cholesterol, which in different tissues may be under
the control of different pituitary hormones, and because
there exists widespread competition of steroids for bind-
ing to receptor sites.

There are many problems associated with the administration of specific hormones. Testosterone, for instance, can cause enlargement of the *prostate gland,* and even stimulate prostate cancer. Estrogen administration can result in a higher incidence of endometrial bleeding and cancer, and over-stimulation of breast tissues possibly leading to a higher incidence of breast cancer. This is because the control mechanisms of these organs and tissues can become overwhelmed when too-high doses of estrogen are given. Progesterone administration concurrent with estrogen therapy reduces the risk of endometrial cancer. If, instead, we give the steroidal precursors, such as DHEA and Preg, tissues and cells can decide how to transform these hormones to be best utilized in the cell in the right proportions. Overstimulation and untoward reactions are less likely.

Thus far, we've discussed giving Preg in combination with DHEA and other sex steroids. It is also possible that Preg and DHEA can be given in combination with other hormones, such as melatonin. As you can see, there's a lot of potential for Preg, but it will take much research to find out how it can be used best.

Dr. Maria Majewska, Ph.D., of the National Institute on

Drug Abuse, Medications Development Division in Rockville, Maryland, says we have to take a new look at hormone replacement. She tells me that perhaps estrogens alone are not the ideal hormones, and that DHEA, possibly in combination with Preg and smaller amounts of estrogens (in women), may be more appropriate.

Why can't a woman be more like a man?

Do you remember this famous line from *My Fair Lady*?

I heard that line as a child and have often pondered it (not that men necessarily have better, or worse, qualities than women—the sexes are just different). During medical school, I learned that female and male brains are not only slightly different anatomically, but are exposed to different amounts of hormones. Men are exposed to more androgens while women are exposed to more estrogens. One fact that people generally don't know, though, is that women do have testosterone in their systems and that testosterone affects not only a woman's brain, but her entire body.

Over the past two or more decades, women have been given estrogen not only for hot flashes, but also as hormone replacement therapy to counteract osteoporosis and to decrease the incidence of heart disease and stroke. Recently, some doctors have started using testosterone replacement in both men and women. There's a 50 percent decline in testosterone levels in women between the ages of 20 and 50 (Zumoff, 1995). Furthermore, the ovaries after menopause stop making testosterone and estrogens. The decline in testosterone levels often leads to impaired sexual function, decreased well-being, loss of energy, and thinning of bones. Therefore, some women are not only taking estrogen pills, but also taking testosterone supplements. In fact, one pharmaceutical company has a combination estrogen and testosterone pill.

Women need male hormones

At the sixth annual meeting of the North American Menopause Society (as reported in *American Family Physician,* Feb. 15, 1996, page 939), there was talk of adding testosterone to the estrogen replacement therapy regimen for women. In one study, 12 women received a daily dose of estrogen (1.25 mg), and 13 women received a daily dose of the same estrogen combined with 2.5 mg of methyltestosterone for nine weeks. Both treatments improved physical symptoms of menopause, such as hot flashes and vaginal dryness, but only the combined regimen significantly relieved psychological symptoms, such as nervousness and irritability. The combined therapy also eased insomnia and fatigue. In another study, Davis and colleagues, researchers from Australia, report, "Testosterone administration to postmenopausal women enhances sexuality and can be of considerable benefit to women experiencing persistently low libido despite adequate estrogen replacement."

Since DHEA is converted into both testosterone and estrogen, could women use DHEA instead of a combination of estrogen and testosterone? In a 1996 article entitled "Androgens and the Postmenopausal Woman," Davis and colleagues raise that very possibility. They say:

> *Androgens [one being testosterone] are important hormones in women and have diverse actions. The decline in the production of ovarian and adrenal androgens and pre-androgens that commences in the decade preceding menopause may impact significantly on women's health. Androgen deficiency in women has only been recently acknowledged, and although still controversial, androgen replacement is becoming an increasingly available option.*

> *The option of androgen replacement should be given to*

*postmenopausal women who suffer persistent loss of well-being, fatigue, and most commonly, loss of libido, despite adequate estrogen replacement and after exclusion of other possible underlying medical conditions. **Treatment with DHEA is potentially an alternative means of replacing androgens in older women.** Future research should clarify the usefulness and safety of this therapy.*

Flory, a 45-year-old patient, tells me, "My sex drive has been gradually going down since my early thirties and for the last few years I've noticed that I pull back when I'm on a date with a guy and he wants to kiss me. I started with 20 mg of DHEA every other day and a month later, I noticed that my urge to be intimate had returned. I now actually enjoy long, intimate kisses."

Having treated many women with DHEA and surveyed a large number who are taking this hormone, I am convinced that a significant number find that they have an improved libido. This is most likely due to DHEA's conversion into testosterone. One patient even told me, "Now that I'm on DHEA, my husband can't keep up with me anymore!" Another female patient recounts, "I feel like a construction worker, but this time eyeing all the men that walk by." I believe that with DHEA many women can regain some of the sexual drive that they had lost over the decades.

The bottom line is that if doctors are planning to use testosterone to replace declining levels of androgens, they should instead seriously consider DHEA. This applies to both men and women.

Should you horse around with estrogens?

Most of the studies conducted in the last few decades concerning the role of estrogen replacement in bone formation, heart health, and cancer have been done using

Premarin. Premarin is the product name of the combination of estrogens (equi-estrogens) obtained from the urine of pregnant mares. Many of these horse estrogens (equilin, equilenin) have chemical configurations different from the estrogens found normally in humans (estriol, estrone, and estradiol). Thus, we don't know the consequences of long-term use of human estrogens in postmenopausal women, and how these consequences would differ from those of horse estrogens. Could the use of human estrogens result in a lower, or higher, rate of uterine or breast cancer? What about the influence on bone formation? Should we administer all three major human estrogens, or just one or two? If we administer all three, . what should be the proportion? Is it better to give pills, creams, or patches? Should one use estrogens continuously or cyclically? With or without progesterone? And most importantly, in what dosages?

The human body is incredibly complicated. Sometimes I wonder if we'll ever adequately answer all these questions. We can only make recommendations based on what we know and sometimes we can only offer an educated guess. That's why you hear a variety of opinions on estrogen replacement. This will continue, I'm sure, for at least another decade or two.

One way to decrease the risk of breast and uterine cancer is to administer a lower dose of estrogens, such as half or two-thirds the normal dose. In one study done by Dr. Morris Notelovitz, director of the Women's Medical and Diagnostic Center in Gainesville, Florida, 0.3 mg of Premarin (instead of 0.625 mg) increased bone mineral density without the risk of endometrial hyperplasia, that is, overgrowth of the uterine lining (Notelovitz, 1996).

Recently, estrogen replacement has been found to increase the rate of blood clotting, resulting in a threefold higher rate of pulmonary embolism or a clot in the lung circulation (Grodstein, 1996). Since DHEA has blood-thinning abilities, could its use partially lessen this risk?

Soy salvation

And then there are the plant estrogens, such as those found in soybeans. At the American Heart Association's 1996 scientific conference, researchers discussed the growing evidence that soybean ingestion may relieve some of the symptoms of menopause. Dr. Gregory Burke, of Bowman Gray School of Medicine in Winston-Salem, North Carolina, reported that women suffering hot flashes had less intense symptoms after ingesting soy protein.

Forty-three women, aged 45 to 55, who suffered daily bouts of hot flashes or night sweats were given 20 grams of powdered soy protein for six weeks. Then they were given 20 grams of powdered carbohydrate for six weeks. The volunteers were not aware until the end of the study whether they were consuming soy protein or carbohydrate.

Although the frequency of hot flashes was not reduced, the severity of the episodes was. The researchers believe the key ingredient of soy protein is phytoestrogen, the plant form of human estrogen. Soy estrogens act on the same chemical targets or receptors in the body that human estrogens affect, although they are less potent. Estimates are that they are 500 to 1,000 times weaker. However, when soy products are eaten, they are consumed in dozens of grams, as opposed to 0.3 to 0.625 mg of regular estrogens. Thus, they could potentially play a significant role in the management of menopausal and postmenopausal symptoms.

Further studies will determine how the increased consumption of tofu, soy milk, and other forms of soybean products reduces the required dosages of estrogen.

Estrogens alone, or a hormone soup?

"I'm already on estrogens, could I add DHEA and Preg to

my regimen?" This is a question I'm asked frequently by patients, at lectures, or while I'm doing radio interviews.

Since DHEA gets partially converted into female hormones, women would probably need to reduce their dose of estrogens. The exact reduction is hard to predict. Could Preg and DHEA supplements eliminate the need for estrogens? I think this is unlikely. Some amount of estrogen in postmenopausal women should be provided. In one small article published over four decades ago, Preg alone was not found be to have significant estrogenic effects (Henderson, 1950). Certainly, more research is needed.

Pondering progesterone

Progesterone itself has a variety of health benefits and should be considered in hormone replacement therapy. It has bone-building properties and prevents the overgrowth of the uterine lining in women on estrogen. Most of the progesterone pills currently prescribed by doctors are the synthetic versions, called progestins. One such progestin is Provera (medroxyprogesterone).

At the American Heart Association's 1996 science conference, Giuseppe Rosano, MD, of the Instituto Scientifico in Milan, Italy, discussed his findings on natural progesterone (JAMA, 1997). He gave natural progesterone to 18 women with coronary artery disease and synthetic progesterone (medroxyprogesterone) to another group. Both groups were already on estrogen replacement. The progesterone was given ten days a month by intravaginal cream.

Women given the natural progesterone fared better. On exercise electrocardiograms, they were found to have better oxygen delivery to the heart muscle than the group on medroxyprogesterone. In fact, many of the women on medroxyprogesterone performed poorly on this treadmill test.

Natural progesterone has a pleasant, mood-elevating effect. I have personally experimented with the sublingual form on several occasions. It has "feel good" qualities similar to Preg, although I've personally enjoyed the feeling on Preg more. Progesterone is currently a prescription hormone, although you can find natural progesterone creams over-the-counter. These creams are legally allowed to contain only small amounts of the hormone. I believe natural progesterone will become more popular unless we find Preg can take its place. Since Preg is easily converted into progesterone (see diagram on page 18) and is now available without a prescription, I suspect it will partially, or even mostly, replace the use of progesterone.

Can Preg replace DHEA, progesterone, and other adrenal hormones?

Since Preg, The Grandmother of All Steroid Hormones, can be converted into DHEA, progesterone and 150 other steroid hormones, why not use it exclusively, to proverbially "kill two birds with one stone"? I think that eventually we'll find that the best hormone replacement regimen involves giving a little bit of Preg, DHEA, and testosterone to men, and Preg, DHEA, and estrogens (and progesterone?) to women. Young people have the ability to easily convert Preg into all the other steroid hormones. As we age, the enzymes that convert Preg to DHEA and Preg to progesterone may not work as well. Nor would the enzymes that convert DHEA into androgens and estrogens be as effective (see diagram on page 18). Therefore, in older individuals, giving Preg alone would not be enough. See Appendix C for a case history that illustrates this in detail.

The psychological antiaging benefits of hormones

When we discuss the antiaging potential of DHEA, Preg,

and other hormones, we often focus on their physical benefits or hazards to the immune system, bones, heart, prostate, breast, and other tissues and organs. We weigh all these possible benefits and risks in order to decide whether replacement should be undertaken. We often fail to take into account the various psychological benefits that are an outcome of the replacement therapy. Positive influences on mood, well-being, energy, motivation, and stress reduction could, by themselves, influence longevity. Consider the following:

- Being more cheerful, peaceful, and pleasant is noticed by others. Our relationships improve with family, friends, children, and coworkers. Better friendships, fewer arguments, and the subsequent deeper relationships are thought to provide a variety of health benefits.

- Enhanced cognitive function leads to quicker learning, better memory, and perhaps even improved creative talents.

- The well-being we experience on Preg allows us to better enjoy life. Visual and auditory experiences are enhanced. Travel, and seeing new sights, can be more thrilling. Being excited about life can help us live longer. It is believed that low mood or depression can accelerate the aging process.

- Another advantage of feeling good is that we no longer have such a compulsion toward bad habits. We may no longer drink excessively, smoke cigarettes, overeat, or engage in other harmful activities generally done in order to raise mood. If you are already feeling good, you don't need to self-medicate as much with harmful substances, such as coffee and high-sugar, high-fat snacks.

- The energy boost that Preg provides can motivate many

to take long walks or other exercise. The outcome is stronger bones, more toned muscles, fewer bone fractures, and an even more enhanced sense of well-being due to the positive effect of exercise on brain chemistry.

As you can see, the psychological benefits of taking DHEA or Preg can have tremendous direct and indirect influences on our physical health and life span. These psychological factors cannot be measured when studies are done with mice. How can a researcher measure the effect of Preg on a mouse's ability to get a job promotion?

Does Preg have a role in hormone replacement therapy in seniors?

James F. Flood, Ph.D., St. Louis University School of Medicine and Veterans Administration Medical Center, Missouri, has studied the effects of Preg on memory in rodents, and offers this opinion:

> *Yes, of course, Preg can be helpful in treating the general malaise that occurs with aging. Seniors have low Preg levels and replacement could lead to more energy, a more positive outlook, and improvement in memory. I prefer people use low doses, such as 2 to 10 mg, until we learn more.*
>
> *My concern with Preg being available over the counter is with young people self-medicating. We have no idea what would happen if people with normal Preg levels take this hormone for very long periods. If young people in their 20s or 30s who have normal Preg levels take excessive amounts of Preg for many years or decades, it could theoretically lead to permanent and irreversible changes in neurotransmitter levels or receptors in their brains, especially on the cholinergic system. Preg may,*

just as alcohol or other drugs do, permanently alter threshold levels of receptors. In fact, some people are never able to quit drinking coffee because many years of daily drinking downregulates caffeine receptors in the brain. This is also true with long-term smoking, which permanently influences nicotine receptors. Long-term use of amphetamines and some diet pills can have a permanent negative effect on dopamine receptors. I think the use of Preg by younger people for short periods of time for a specific medical or psychological condition would be okay and not lead to any irreversible neurochemical changes.

I can't foresee any health problems or untoward changes in brain chemistry when older individuals who are lacking adequate amounts of this hormone use low replacement doses under a physician's guidance.

John Morley, M.D., Professor of Medicine, Division of Geriatrics, St. Louis University, Missouri, researches the clinical aspects of Preg:

Our knowledge of Preg is in its infancy. However, based on the human studies on Preg over the past few decades, plus the existing animal studies, I think there clearly seems to be a place for Preg replacement for many older people. We're currently conducting some studies with Preg administration to seniors.

We're not at the stage to recommend it clinically, though, since we need more data. I don't like the fact that it's available over the counter. There's a great deal we don't know about Preg's properties. However, if a doctor were to prescribe Preg, my personal opinion is that I think it would be more appropriate than prescribing DHEA since Preg is converted into DHEA.

Summary

I believe that with the right mix of hormone supplements, we can improve the quality of our lives, as well as hopefully make them longer. The trick is to find the right combination. How do we know which to take and how much?

It's very difficult to say. It will take us decades to learn the long-term effects of different hormone supplements and their combinations. In the meantime, many of these hormones are easily available and the public wants answers. One way to get an idea on how much you need is to get blood tests for hormone levels, including Preg, progesterone, DHEA, estrogens, testosterone, melatonin, and other hormones. If those levels are low, supplements could be appropriate. If you can afford this, or your insurance pays for it, and you find a health care provider who has experience interpreting the values, this information could prove useful.

We must realize, however, that even if we know what our bloodstream hormone levels are, we don't know for sure what the levels are where it really counts; in tissues and cells. There are different enzymes in tissues that metabolize hormones in different ways. For instance, prostate tissue could metabolize DHEA and Preg differently than brain tissue. Ovarian tissue could metabolize these hormones differently than breast tissue. There are advantages and disadvantages to testing that we'll discuss in Chapter 10.

Another approach is to take low doses of a hormone, become accustomed to how that feels, and then gradually add another, monitoring one's mood, energy, sleep, and well-being. Doing this in a careful and logical way could possibly bypass the need for extensive testing.

In view of our limited knowledge about Preg and other hormones, I cannot give any definite recommendations regarding long-term replacement. However, in Chapter 9, I will provide some useful guidelines.

In the following chapters, we'll look at long-ignored studies on how Preg can help us deal with the effects of stress, as well as how it influences the rest of our bodies.

CHAPTER 5

LESS STRESS

Without a doubt, stress can profoundly influence the rate at which our brain cells age and become damaged. There is a special area in the brain called the hippocampus, which is involved in memory storage. This area actually shrinks when the brain is exposed to too high a dose of stress hormones. Stress affects not only our brain cells, but also the rest of the cells of our body. Mind you, a little stress is healthy because it challenges our brain and body to perform better. However, if it becomes excessive, there comes a point where our organs become exhausted and breakdowns can occur.

Stress is known to alter the amount and type of steroid hormones produced. This can lead to a failure in the maintenance of ideal hormonal balances. An excess of cortisol is produced, which has significant negative consequences. The end result may lead to mental and physical diseases.

Excess cortisol has a variety of harmful effects, including increases in blood sugar levels. High amounts of cortisol also inhibit the immune system and cause calcium loss, leading to osteoporosis.

In fact, excess cortisol, by crippling the immune system, increases the rate of infections. Processes that repair tissues can be shut down; sleep is interfered with; bones can become osteoporotic; and there could even be an increase in cancer risk. Certain cancers, cervical cancer for example, are partly caused by the human papilloma virus. Since stress interferes with the immune system, virus-causing cancers could get a foothold and start growing at a rapid rate.

Even though, as a rule, most of us are not involved in demanding physical labor, we are exposed to an enormous amount of psychological stress. We drive to work in the morning in horn-honking heavy traffic, followed by work tensions involving difficult bosses, deadlines, phone calls to return, and projects to complete. We have the traffic again on the way back home; dinner to prepare; overactive children to keep under control, feed, and nurture; bills to pay; and a home and garden to maintain. Sometimes, there are social conflicts: disputes with relatives, friends, and loved ones. To add further insult, some unfortunate souls can't even get enough hours of restful sleep, and are therefore still stunned in the morning when the alarm clock prematurely blares the onset of another hectic day. It's enough to make our adrenal glands cry, "Uncle!"

Can Preg come to the rescue?

The use of Preg, by itself or in combination with DHEA, has the potential to decrease the harmful effects of excess cortisol and stress.

It has been known for some time that when people are under stress, the adrenal glands make more steroid hormones. There comes a point, though, that the adrenal glands get tired and can't produce as many of these steroids. At this point, a person starts feeling fatigue.

Back in 1945, 97 healthy young workers in industrial factories received 50 mg of Preg per day. The study included 8 leather cutters, 12 lathe operators, and 77 optical workers. These workers were engaged in a variety of operations involving incentive piecework, so the more they produced, the more they got paid. Preg administration improved production rates. These workers felt less fatigued and were better able to cope with their jobs. They also reported a sense of well-being. Drs. Pincus and Hoagland, who conducted the study, wrote:

> *We are convinced that Preg is most effective in combating fatigue where motivation is high and where men are working under really trying conditions. There were no untoward side effects.*

One of the most remarkable attributes of this hormone is its ability to provide a balancing, or harmonizing, feeling. Users often note a calm, peaceful disposition with the ability to ward off fatigue. One 52-year-old female patient told me, "When I take Preg I feel more balanced and organized. There are no ups and downs. I feel steady, on an even plateau, and harmonious with others and myself. 'Centered and peaceful' are other words that I would use. There is a slight energy that comes on. I guess the word 'well-being' is another good one."

There may be a neurochemical reason for this peaceful feeling. Dr. Wu, from the Department of Pharmacology and Experimental Therapeutics at Boston University School of Medicine, has studied the role of Preg on brain cells. He says, "Our observations are consistent with the hypothesis that neurosteroids such as pregnenolone sulfate are involved in regulating the balance between excitation and inhibition in the central nervous system."

I wonder if this partially explains the balanced and harmonious feeling people have while on Preg.

Resurrecting long-buried studies

Back in 1944, Dr. Hudson Hoagland, Executive Director of the Worcester Foundation for Experimental Biology in Massachusetts, studied the effects of stress on the output of adrenal steroids. Aviators were exposed to many hours of experiments that simulated the operation of an airplane in flight. This obviously led to psychological fatigue. The amount of adrenal steroids produced was determined by measuring the quantity of adrenal steroid metabolites in the urine (called 17-ketosteroids). The stress of the experiment dramatically increased the production of adrenal steroids as measured by urinary 17-ketosteroids. When Dr. Hoagland gave them 50 mg of Preg, he found their performance was enhanced and the increase in adrenal 17-ketosteroids was lessened (Hoagland, 1944). The volunteers mentioned they felt less fatigued. He reports, "This we believe indicates a sparing action of hormone secretion on the adrenal cortex when Preg is administered." Interestingly, no effect was seen in diminishing fatigue or stress when another hormone, progesterone, was given. Adrenal cortex extracts were also found to be ineffective.

Levels of steroid hormones in the brain respond quickly when exposed to stress. An acute stress, such as carbon dioxide inhalation or electric foot shock, elicited a marked increase in the concentrations of Preg, progesterone, and corticosterone in the brains of laboratory rats (Barbaccia, 1994). The researchers say, "These data show that the rat brain cortical and hippocampal steroid content is related to the emotional state of the animal." It's possible that the human brain would also respond to stress by making more Preg, but there may come a time where chronic stress may exhaust the ability of the brain to maintain the high levels of steroid hormones. This would lead to mental exhaustion.

Preg and the stresses of daily life

No matter what your occupation, you may find that Preg can help you cope with the stresses of the workplace by helping you become more even tempered and alert, and by making it easier to take a more positive attitude. This would allow you to deal more constructively with what happens in your work environment. Whether you are someone who works in a high stress environment (such as a hospital worker, firefighter, or police officer) or someone who works in an environment filled with more subtle stresses (such as an accountant, lawyer, or secretarial worker), you may find Preg beneficial when used on an occasional basis.

Of course, the workplace is not the only source of stress for many people. There are many stresses in the social environment. If you are married, you may be dealing with problems in your marriage. If you are a parent, you may be having trouble with your children. If you are single, you may be coping with loneliness. Or you may be dealing with stress from other sources, such as the aftereffects of violent crime. Again, Preg used on an occasional basis may help you find the mental peace you need to effectively cope with such situations.

You should also take advantage of other stress-reducing therapies, such as exercise, meditation, yoga, biofeedback, and others. Preg can be used in combination with these modalities. I've enjoyed my yoga sessions while on Preg.

One caution to note: certain individuals may find that high doses of Preg induce irritability or impatience, leading to an aggressive attitude or snapping remarks. Make sure you have experimented with a variety of doses and forms of Preg, and know how you react to it before you take a high dose on a particularly stressful day.

Melatonin is an additional supplement that can relieve stress in those who have insomnia. This hormone should be seriously considered for occasional use to provide a deeper and fuller sleep. As we all know, a restful, long and uninterrupted night of slumber can do wonders in making us feel refreshed and ready to face the day with renewed enthusiasm and a smile. For more details on how to use this hormone appropriately, see *Melatonin: Nature's Sleeping Pill*. Your dose should be low, such as 0.1 mg to 1 mg. Higher doses can lead to next day tiredness and excessive dreaming.

Whenever I've taken Preg and then gone on a long walk or hike in the mountains, I've noticed that I'm less fatigued. This makes me wonder whether Preg could be useful for those who engage in demanding physical activities, such as mountain climbing, or other strenuous outdoor activities.

CHAPTER 6

ARTHRITIS AND AUTOIMMUNE CONDITIONS

There are several rheumatological conditions—conditions that primarily affect the joints, muscles, bones, and nerves—for which Preg can be beneficial, either by itself, or most likely, in combination with other therapies and medicines. These conditions include ankylosing spondylitis, lupus, two forms of arthritis, and scleroderma.

Ankylosing spondylitis (AS)

AS is a chronic inflammatory disease of the joints in the spine that leads to back pain and stiffening. The age of onset is usually in the late teens or early 20s. The incidence is greater in males. The standard medical therapy is the use of NSAIDs (non-steroidal anti-inflammatory drugs).

In one study done in the 1940s, researchers found that the use of Preg led to marked clinical improvement in patients with AS (Davison, 1947; McGavack, 1951). Full details as to dosages were not provided in the article, but they generally ranged between 50 mg and 100 mg.

Lupus

Systemic lupus erythematosus (SLE) is an *autoimmune* condition four times as common in women as in men. Symptoms include painful and swollen joints, skin rash, and mouth ulcers. A special blood test, called the antinuclear antibody test, is used for diagnosis.

Eleven women with lupus between the ages of 24 and 51 were given Preg. As a rule, after three days of therapy, they experienced a sense of well-being (McGavack, 1951). In many of the treated patients, there was improvement in joint pain and a marked reduction in skin rash. One 24-year-old patient had suffered from a skin rash and joint pains for seven years. After the third day of treatment, her joint pains subsided, her appetite improved, and her skin rash began to recede. Three weeks later, her sedimentation rate dropped from 160 to 80 mm, indicating an abatement of her disease.

DHEA has also been found to be helpful in lupus. The possibility of using a combination of Preg and DHEA should be explored.

Even if Preg and DHEA are not found to be curative on their own, they should be tested in combination with other forms of medical therapy.

Osteoarthritis

Osteoarthritis is a degenerative disease of joints estimated to affect more than 30 million Americans. It is the most common chronic condition.

Back in 1951, McGavack and colleagues gave 13 patients with osteoarthritis injections of Preg, with dosages ranging between 50 and 200 mg. Seven of the patients showed a moderate or marked improvement while six obtained little or no benefit. A sense of well-being and increased appetite were commonly experienced within two to four days after starting treatment. Within five to eight days, pain decreased and the range of motion of the joints increased. Patients who were bedridden started walking in 10 to 14 days. After four to five weeks of gradual improvement, the disease symptoms could not be further influenced, regardless of dose. Upon cessation of therapy, joint pains usually returned. Temperature, white blood cell count, and sedimentation rates were unaffected by the therapy.

Dr. Arnold Fox, a physician in private practice in Beverly Hills, California, says:

> *I remember Preg from the 1950s, when it was mentioned in medical school as a form of therapy for arthritis. Preg, at that time, was being sold without a prescription. But then cortisone came on the scene and that changed everything—Preg use went down the drain. Cortisone gave remarkable short-term improvements but then later we learned about its terrible side effects, including immune suppression and osteoporosis.*
>
> *I'm currently taking Preg as part of an overall anti-aging process. I'm taking it in combination with DHEA and other supplements such as antioxidants. I think Preg should be part of the program in older individuals since it helps with memory. Preg has been around a long time—it has stood the test of time. As far as arthritis is concerned, it helped people back in the 50s and now we're coming back to it. One additional benefit to the use of Preg is that it makes people feel better.*

A variety of nutrients have a role to pay in osteoarthritis. One nutrient that has shown enormous promise is glucosamine, generally in a dose of 500 mg three times a day.

Rheumatoid Arthritis

Back in 1950, researchers gave 300 mg of Preg daily for 40 days to patients suffering from rheumatoid arthritis (Henderson, 1950). They report:

The first improvement noted was absence of pain on motion and disappearance of tenderness. Absence of pain on motion permits greater joint mobility, which in turn leads to less spasticity and greater muscular strength. The patient who responds to Preg therapy is usually able within a few days to perform muscular action impossible in previous months, or even years, such as dressing, stooping to tie shoes, combing hair, sitting and rising, lying and rising, raising arms above the head and lowering them slowly ... climbing and descending stairs ....

In another study, 21 patients received injections of 100 mg of Preg acetate for five to thirty days, followed by 100 mg one to three times weekly. Five did not improve, four improved slightly, four benefited moderately, and eight patients showed marked improvement (Henderson, 1950). The researchers conclude:

Preg is a steroid having pharmacological and hormonal behavior which has not been satisfactorily characterized within any familiar framework. A fair proportion of rheumatoid arthritics receiving Preg in sufficient dosage for an adequate period show symptomatic changes sufficiently favorable to warrant further study. The substance has an extraordinarily low order of toxicity. Its properties are diverse, and somewhat obscure, and seem intriguing enough to encourage further inquiry.

Another study was published by Dr. Harry Freeman and colleagues from the Worcester Foundation for Experimental Biology in Shrewsbury, Massachusetts. The study included 62 patients—17 men and 45 women. The average age of the patients was 48 years and most had suffered from rheumatoid arthritis for 10 years. Five hundred mg of Preg was given daily to each patient for a period of two to 30 weeks. Twenty-four patients experienced striking improvement, 20 showed minor improvement and 14 showed no improvement. There was a tendency to relapse when the medication was discontinued. There was also a direct relationship between the length of time Preg was administered and the length of time improvement was maintained after the medication was stopped (Freeman, 1950).

In some cases, when improvement did not occur in two weeks, the dose of Preg was increased to 800 mg. However, this high dose did not cause any further improvement.

It remains to be seen how Preg can be effectively used in combination with other currently prescribed medicines to alleviate the pain and other symptoms of rheumatoid arthritis. Preg does not appear to be curative, but has the potential to be effectively used in combination with other medicines such as NSAIDs, and perhaps even gold, methotrexate, and other drugs. Most NSAIDs have significant side effects, including stomach ulcers and kidney damage, that limit their usefulness. If low doses of Preg are found to be effective in combination with NSAIDs, their dosages could be lowered, thus minimizing untoward reactions.

Annette Stoesser, M.D., from Roswell, New Mexico, tells me: "I generally use Preg in my patients for memory and energy improvement. I've used high doses, such as 100 mg for rheumatoid arthritis in three women with some benefits, including less swelling. Major complaints that patients have noticed on high doses include agitation and overstimulation." For more dosage information, see Chapter 9.

Scleroderma

Also called progressive systemic sclerosis, this condition consists of hardening and rigidity of the skin, and even fibrosis of some internal organs. Early manifestations are aches in the joints and Raynaud's phenomenon (spasms of blood vessels in fingers in response to cold or emotional stress). The causes of scleroderma are not known, but autoimmunity, abnormalities of fibroblasts (certain cells of connective tissue), and occupational exposure to silica are thought to play a role. Symptoms usually appear between ages 30 and 50, and women are affected two to three times as commonly as men are.

Two women with scleroderma, ages 56 and 65, were given about 100 mg of Preg (McGavack, 1951). By the end of the first week, there was softening of the skin over the face, forearms, and hands. Improvement in the texture and elasticity of the skin continued for the first five weeks of therapy, after which no further progress in the softening process occurred. The improvement that had already been achieved was maintained.

It would be interesting to experiment using creams containing Preg on a variety of skin disorders, including wrinkles, hair disorders, psoriasis, scleroderma, and others.

How does Preg work in arthritic disorders?

In 1951, Dr. McGavack and colleagues, in an article entitled "The use of pregnenolone in various clinical disorders," conclude:

> The behavior of pregnenolone in our cases of rheumatoid arthritis, osteoarthritis, Still's disease [a juvenile form of chronic arthritis], acute arthritis, exophtalmos [bulging eyes associated with thyroid disease], and gout leads us to the conclusion that benefit, when obtained, has shown some degree of relationship which is usually directly proportional to the amount of active inflammatory reaction. In other words, long-standing articular and periarticular [tendons, tissues, muscles, and ligaments near joints] lesions are less susceptible to a favorable influence than the lesions of recent and obviously inflammatory nature. For instance, in osteoarthritis the

joint lesion itself is one of little or no inflammatory reaction. In these cases, most, if not all of the changes we have observed have occurred in the periarticular lesions, such as the fibrositis and myositis.

Dr. McGavack noted the earliest clinical changes to be between the third and the seventh days after therapy was started. A sense of well-being and an increased appetite were the first responses to pregnenolone. These effects might often appear before there were any noticeable alterations in the joint pains or other clinical manifestations. With improvement in pain, joint mobility was increased, active motion encouraged, and muscular atrophy reduced. There was a definite tendency for joint symptoms to recur when therapy was stopped, but starting the treatment again proved beneficial. The researchers suggest several possible theories for these improvements:

● The effect of Preg on pituitary gland hormones

● Preg's conversion to progesterone and other hormones, including cortisol

● Its direct effects on a variety of tissues including capillaries and the supporting matrix of skin and mucous membranes. They believe this is the most likely possibility.

Dr. McGavack and his colleagues go on: "The ability of pregnenolone to affect the tissues beneficially in chronic lupus, scleroderma, and malignant exophtalmos was in most instances striking."

Summary

Preg's potential in helping arthritic conditions has not been fully realized and we should revive scientific interest in this hormone. I think the greatest benefit we'll find with Preg is its use in combination with other nutrients and medicines. I caution users and physicians to stay with low doses. Take high doses only for brief periods of time.

CHAPTER 7

NEUROLOGICAL HELP

Preg is made in neural tissues, including the brain and peripheral nervous system (the nerves beyond the brain and spinal cord). It makes sense that it would play a role in a variety of neurological conditions. However, we know very little of what it actually does and in which conditions supplementation would prove beneficial. This whole field is wide open for exploration and I'm eager to find out what future research will discover.

Alzheimer's disease (AD)

The cause of this feared mental deterioration is not fully known. A patient with this condition starts losing memory and the ability to think clearly, and, eventually, cannot even recognize loved family members. Interestingly, indomethacin, a nonsteroidal anti-inflammatory drug similar to aspirin, has been found to be helpful with this condition. This indicates that AD may involve, at least partially, an inflammatory process. However, the side effects of gastrointestinal discomfort and potential stomach ulcers limit the therapeutic potential of indomethacin.

Dr. Flood believes Preg plays a role in AD. He tells me, "Preg can act on *glutamate* receptors and the cholinergic system [the nerve impulse transportation system for acetylcholine]. This hormone could be useful in conditions where the cholinergic system of the brain is not functioning well. Alzheimer's disease is one such condition where cholinergic replacement could be beneficial."

In 1995, Dr. Roberts tried giving 525 mg of Preg per day to 20 patients with AD. Unfortunately, no benefits were found. Dr. Roberts believes that 525 mg was too high, and was counterproductive due to side effects. Perhaps a lower dosage would have been more appropriate. For dosage information, see Chapter 9.

Multiple sclerosis (MS)

MS is a disease of the central nervous system that occurs most commonly in young or middle adulthood. The cause is not fully known, but some researchers think it involves a T-cell mediated autoimmune process. Exposure to certain viral infections in childhood may be a causative factor. Acute attacks could also be triggered by viral infections. It is believed that environmental factors, such as common viruses, act early in life in people with a genetic predisposition.

In MS, the sheath (myelin) that surrounds certain nerves breaks down. The destruction of this sheath is known as demyelination. Common symptoms include unsteadiness, loss of muscular coordination, weakness, speech difficulties and rapid involuntary movements of the eyes.

There's a certain type of cell that surrounds nerves to form this sheath or myelin. These cells are called Schwann cells, named after the 19th century German physician who discovered them. Interestingly, Schwann cells have been found to contain large concentrations of both Preg and DHEA (Morfin, 1992). It is now thought that nerve cells in the peripheral nervous system produce Preg and DHEA. We also know that certain cells called oligodendrocytes also make these steroids in the brain (the central nervous system).

Based on the fact that Preg and DHEA are made in nerves, and that MS is a condition involving the breakdown of the sheath surrounding these nerves, it was thought that DHEA might reduce MS symptoms.

Nine female and 12 male patients with MS were given 90 mg of DHEA each day for 14 weeks (Roberts, 1990). Three of the women and seven of the men reported feeling more energetic and that their quality of life had improved. However, there were no apparent improvements in their neurological symptoms.

One of the problems with high-dose DHEA is that it is virilizing or masculinizing. Women can quickly develop fine facial hair or acne. Dr. Roberts believes that a combination of Preg and DHEA might lessen this problem. In his 1995 article, he says, "A combination of Preg and small doses of DHEA might show a synergistic effect in relieving fatigue in MS without virilization."

Also in 1995, scientists discovered that both progesterone and its precursor, Preg, are significantly involved in the healing process of damaged nerves. In a study done at the University of Bordeaux in Talence, France, the sciatic nerves of rats were cut. (The sciatic nerves are two large bundles of nerves that start at the lower end of our spinal column and go through our buttocks on each side. They branch out into muscles and tissues of our thighs and legs.) When the local production of progesterone or Preg was inhibited, the myelin sheaths did not form around the repaired nerves. When Preg and progesterone were administered, the myelin sheaths formed normally (Koenig, 1995).

There are no fully successful medical therapies for MS at this time. Some therapies currently used include short courses of synthetic corticosteroids, genetically engineered immunomodulators such as interferon beta-1b, interferon beta-1a, and the use of copolymer-1, which is made up of glutamic acid, lysine, alanine and tyrosine (Brod, 1996). See Chapter 9 for Preg dosage information.

Nerve injuries

It is possible that Preg could prove useful for those who have suffered nerve injuries due to accidents, burns, or electrical shock. In one study, rats with damaged spinal cords were treated with a combination of indomethacin, an anti-inflammatory drug, and Preg (Guth, 1994). This treatment reduced damage to nerve cells and increased restoration of activity. Amazingly, 11 of 16 of the rats treated with this combination were able to stand and walk at 21 days after the injury, four of them almost normally. The results were far superior to those obtained in *controls* or in animals to which the substances were given separately. The researchers conclude, "This approach may prove to be applicable to nervous system injury, in general, and to injury in other tissues."

Parkinson's disease (PD)

Parkinson's disease is caused by deterioration of a certain brain region know as the substantia nigra. It results in muscle tremors and rigidity, a masklike facial expression, stooped posture, and a shuffling gait. PD, in a minority of cases, is thought to have a genetic component. Preg, because of its positive effects on the brain, should be tested in PD patients. Interestingly, in a German study, researchers found that patients with PD ate significantly fewer vegetables, but more sweets, snacks, raw meat, and organ meats than people without the disease (*Neurology* 47:636–650, 1996). Increasing antioxidant intake through consumption of vegetables, fruits, grains, and other healthy foods is recommended in order to protect brain cells from damage. See Chapter 9 for Preg dosage information.

Seizures

A number of receptors and brain chemicals are involved in seizure promotion or inhibition. Preg influences a variety of receptors. It stimulates NMDA receptors in the brain (Wu, 1991; Maione, 1992) and has both stimulatory and inhibitory effects on GABA receptors. There is ample theoretical reasoning that it could influence seizures. However, we have no human studies to confirm whether it has a helpful or deleterious influence.

I do, though, have an interesting case history. In March 1997, our research center received a call from Pat, a 57-year-old woman from Westminster, Colorado, who has suffered from a seizure disorder since age three. She related to us her interesting medical history:

> *For the last 54 years of my life I've had chronic seizures and doctors have had me on Librium, Valium, Equanil, and every anti-seizure medicine they could think of. I'm currently on Tegretol, Dilantin, phenobarbital, Klonopin, and Synthroid, but I still get a few seizures a day. I can't leave home. I wonder throughout the day when the next one is going to come. My doctors have practically given up on me.*

> *I saw a naturopathic doctor who recommended I try Preg. I had nothing to lose; life can be terrible when you can't leave home. An amazing thing has happened since I started Preg. For the past two months, I've only had three days of seizures. I'm so happy I could jump for joy. I've also noticed that I'm more alert and aware.*

We were intrigued by Pat's story, and called her doctor. Joe Cardot, N.D., who has a practice in Arvada, Colorado, told me, "She's on about 50 mg of Preg and her seizure frequency has dramatically decreased." Dr. Cardot added, "I've also given Preg to a few other patients with petit mal seizures and found it to be beneficial. Furthermore, women with PMS tell me ther their symptoms are improved when they use Preg."

One anecdote means little. I would caution anyone with a seizure disorder who plans to try Preg to do so under extremely close medical supervision. It's possible Preg may make another person's seizure worse. Be supervised.

CHAPTER 8

THE ALL-PURPOSE HORMONE

Hormones have the ability to enter a variety of cells, go to the nucleus, influence certain genes, and cause changes within cells in terms of the formation of new proteins, peptides, and enzymes. Therefore, it is no surprise that taking Preg or other steroid hormones will have an influence on almost all body tissues, including skin, muscle, nerve, heart, and others.

It's a shame that even though we've known about Preg for a few decades, so little research has been done with it. Preg is a natural hormone that cannot be patented. If it weren't for our biomedical research financing system that requires a company to patent a molecule in order to profit from it, we could have been far, far ahead in our understanding of the therapeutic potential of this fascinating hormone.

Let's discuss a few conditions in which Preg could play a role.

Addison's disease (AD)

AD is an uncommon disorder caused by destruction of the adrenal cortex, the outer portion of the adrenal gland. This leads to deficiencies in cortisol, aldosterone, and adrenal androgens and estrogens. In the United States, autoimmune destruction of the adrenals is the most common cause of AD. Other causes include metastatic carcinoma, infections (such as HIV, tuberculosis, fungal infections), scleroderma, and amyloid disease *(Current Medical Diagnosis and Treatment*, 1997).

Common signs and symptoms of AD include weakness, weight loss, anxiety, and mental irritability. Patients tend to have low blood sugar and low blood pressure. The accepted therapy for AD is replacement with 15 to 25 mg of hydrocortisone, along with mineralocorticoids such as aldosterone.

Six patients with AD were given Preg for periods of time ranging from four to 167 days. Four of the patients were women and two were men (McGavack, 1951). Their ages ranged from 26 to 58 years. The clinical condition of five of these patients was unchanged by Preg, and one individual showed a slight improvement in strength and vigor. Thus it appears that Preg, by itself, is of limited usefulness in AD. However, Preg and DHEA should certainly be further tested, in combination with hydrocortisone and aldosterone, because perhaps they can harmoniously provide some additional adrenal hormones that are deficient. Since autoimmune diseases are a major cause of AD, Preg and DHEA could provide a double benefit since they seem to improve such conditions.

Cancer

The role of Preg in tumor initiation or prevention is largely unknown.

My emphasis in this book is for Preg to be used temporarily, except in cases where doctors are using it as hormone replacement therapy. We don't have any data at this time on the long-term consequences of Preg use. It's possible that it could help prevent some cancers. It's also possible the opposite response may occur. Chances are that low doses, such as 5 or 10 mg, would not be of any significant clinical concern, and could even be beneficial. I certainly don't believe the occasional or temporary use of Preg would have any significant influence on cancer prevention or initiation.

Chronic fatigue syndrome (CFS)

As discussed previously in Chapter 2, Preg was initially found to be useful in relieving fatigue. So there is some theoretical justification in trying Preg for CFS. We should realize, though, that chronic fatigue may have multiple causes that include viruses and depression. A combination of Preg and other nutrients might prove to be a worthy area to explore.

Cholesterol

Some prescription drugs given to patients with high cholesterol levels act by inhibiting the formation of an enzyme called HMGCoA reductase, which is involved in making cholesterol in the body. These medications lower cholesterol levels by inhibiting its formation. However, in doing so, the amount of Preg made is also lowered, leading to impaired brain function. Two of these medications are Pravachol (provastatin) and Mevacor (lovastatin). It is possible that long-term use of these drugs may cause depression, suicide, or violent behavior. There are even suggestions that these drugs can promote certain cancers. Drs. Flood, Morley, and Roberts, in a 1992 article, report, "Low serum levels of pregnenolone in aging and the increases of cancer and behavioral disorders in individuals receiving drugs that block synthesis of cholesterol, the immediate precursor of pregnenolone, suggest possible clinical utility for pregnenolone."

Thus, in order to counteract these negative consequences, it may be worth exploring the possibility of administrating Preg simultaneously with these drugs. This way cholesterol synthesis is blocked, but the rest of the pathways that link Preg to progesterone, and Preg to DHEA and androgens/estrogens, would continue to function.

However, the administration of Preg may not solve the whole problem because cholesterol itself is used in the brain for certain functions. At the National Institute of Health and Medical Research in Paris, Dr. Mahmoud Zureik studied 6,728 men over a 17-year period. In that time, 32 of the men committed suicide. Men with below-average levels of blood cholesterol were three times more likely to kill themselves than those men with average levels (Zureik, 1996).

Diabetes

The relationship of Preg to blood sugar and its influence on insulin are not currently known. I suspect that a low dose, such as 10 mg, would not significantly influence blood sugar levels.

Interestingly, consumption of cow's milk in infancy may be a trigger for the later development of diabetes (Cavallo, 1996). The casein protein in cow's milk may trigger an autoimmune response that can also attack and destroy pancreatic cells. Shouldn't we be feeding infants mother's milk, and if we do feed them cow's milk, should we do so in smaller amounts and partially substitute soy milk?

Heart disease

We know very little on how Preg influences the heart. It may have beneficial effects if used in the right dose. Let's keep in mind that the pacemakers and conduction system of the heart are made of neural tissue and Preg has an influence on neural tissues.

Anecdotally, too-high dosages could aggravate heart irregularities. There are no formal studies that have evaluated the use of Preg in heart disease.

Immune system

No formal studies of the effect of Preg on the human immune system have been published. However, we know that DHEA, one of the metabolites of Preg, can improve the immune system (see *DHEA: A Practical Guide*). In one small study done on mice, it was found that Preg and DHEA are involved in immunity (Morfin, 1994). The researchers state, "Our results suggest that in tissues where immune response takes place, the locally-produced metabolites of Preg and DHEA are involved in a process which may participate in the physiological regulation of the body's immune system."

The immune system is very complicated and at this point we don't know for sure how taking Preg can influence it, and whether Preg will be found to be useful for those with AIDS or other immune system disorders.

Muscle building

DHEA has mild to moderate anabolic (muscle-building) properties. I suspect that Preg's anabolic effects, if any, would be less than those of DHEA.

Postpartum depression

Some women experience a temporary lowering of mood after delivery. A new study shows that there is a connection between falling cholesterol levels and postpartum depression (Ploeckinger, 1996). Twenty healthy women underwent psychiatric interviews and measurements of cholesterol before and after pregnancy. The Austrian researchers found no relationship between absolute cholesterol and mood scores, but did find that a fall in cholesterol levels was strongly associated with poor mood scores. Could this fall lead to a decrease in Preg production?

It would be worthwhile to try Preg in women experiencing postpartum depression, except for those who are breastfeeding. We don't know if Preg can cross into breast milk and, if it does, how it would influence the baby.

Premenstrual syndrome (PMS)

PMS occurs, to some degree, in one third of women of childbearing age. Symptoms include irritability, increased aggressiveness, cravings for sweet or salty foods, nervousness, mood swings, difficulty in concentrating, fatigue, tenderness of the breasts, and abdominal bloating (*Principles of Ambulatory Medicine*, 1991).

These symptoms appear during the latter half of the menstrual cycle and disappear with the onset of menstruation. The exact causes of PMS are not fully known, but hormonal imbalances or "abnormal" responses to the fluctuating hormonal levels (such as progesterone) during the late part of the menstrual cycle are thought to be involved. In a double-blind, randomized, crossover trial, 300 mg of oral micronized progesterone was given for two months to 23 women. The volunteers received the progesterone three days after ovulation up to the beginning of menses. Improvements were noted in anxiety, depression, and stress, and in the physical complaints of swelling and hot flashes (Dennerstein, 1985).

Since Preg is converted into progesterone, could it play a role in PMS? Although no formal studies have been done on the use of Preg for PMS, a few users have noted symptom reduction. Holly, age 29, from Petaluma, California, tells me, "For the last three months I've been experimenting with Preg. At the end of my period, I start with 5 mg daily up to the time of ovulation, and then I gradually increase my dose to 30 mg daily up to the start of my next period. My PMS symptoms are definitely reduced."

Sharon, a 43-year-old psychotherapist from Agoura, California, relates:

> *I've had PMS all my young adult life. I'm now 43 and two weeks of every month I'm miserable and depressed. I've been to traditional doctors and I've also tried homeopathy, acupuncture, thyroid medicines, progesterone cream, herbs, vitamins, and relaxation techniques—all to no avail.*
>
> *This month my symptoms started again, but this time I took 10 mg of Preg. I feel like a normal human being again. I've had no compulsive cravings for sugar and no depression or irritability. My brain feels like it's been scrubbed and cleaned. Most interesting was the visual enhancement— colors are brighter, everything is clearer, sharper, truer—like seeing things for the first time.*

Exercise is also known to reduce PMS symptoms.

I am currently conducting research with the Southwest College of Naturopathic Medicine in Tempe, Arizona, to evaluate the role of Preg in PMS.

Prostate gland

What would happen if patients with prostate enlargement were given Preg? At this point we don't have any studies to tell us whether this hormone would be helpful or harmful. We know testosterone can simulate prostate growtrh. However, Preg supplements, except in very high dosages, are not likely to be metabolized all the way to testosterone.

Skin

Acne—DHEA is known to have strong androgenic (masculinizing) effects and acne is a common feature of high-dose intake. Preg is not as androgenic, and much higher doses are required to induce pimple formation.

Psoriasis—Itchy and reddish patches that can involve either a few areas of the body or, in severe cases, include the arms, legs, scalp, abdomen, and back characterize this skin condition.

Three male patients with psoriasis were treated with an average dose of 60 to 250 mg of Preg. One patient improved but there were no changes in the other two (McGavack, 1951).

Some studies have shown that ingesting more fish oils can be beneficial in psoriasis.

Wrinkles—Dr. Thomas Sternberg and colleagues from the Division of Dermatology, University of California Medical Center, did extensive studies with Preg more than four decades ago. In a 1961 article, they report, "Our interest in pregnenolone dates back to 1950, at which time we administered large doses orally to patients with chronic skin disease, and also used 3 to 6 per cent pregnenolone ointment topically. This study was completely negative insofar as therapeutic effect was concerned and, like other investigators, we found no toxic effects and no evidence of percutaneous [skin] absorption as might be reflected in altered physiological processes."

The researchers became interested in Preg again when other investigators found that topical Preg had hydrating, or moisturizing, effects. They then performed a double-blind study to evaluate the hydrating effects of 0.5 percent Preg in a cream base when used in a group of 86 middle-aged to elderly females exhibiting wrinkling and other signs of skin aging. The creams were applied to one side of the face.

By the third week of the experiment, there was a clear improvement to one side of the face. This improvement continued during the three-month duration of the study. The researchers observed more hydration, fullness, and less wrinkling. When the code was broken at the end of the study, it was the side of the face getting the Preg cream that had improved.

There were three patients who did not tolerate the cream. All three previously had oily skin, seborrheic dermatitis, or acne.

Therefore, it appears that Preg, in a cream or ointment form, should be explored as a way to reverse wrinkling in middle-aged and older individuals.

Substance use disorders

Roger, a 50-year-old from Silver Spring, Maryland, tells me, "I want to thank you, Dr. Sahelian, because I'm taking Preg because of your writings. Preg cut my appetite dramatically and has strongly reduced any desire for alcohol, caffeine, and chocolate. The feeling of well-being seems to make one not want these things anymore."

One of the common reasons people overuse or misuse substances such as alcohol, caffeine, psychoactive drugs, and even chocolate and food, is because they are trying to elevate their mood. Many self-medicate with the best substance they can find. Since Preg elevates mood, it would be worthwhile to conduct studies involving individuals who are prone to substance misuse.

Alcohol withdrawal is the term used when alcoholics suddenly stop their drinking. Withdrawal symptoms include anxiety and depression. Doctors treat these patients with Valium and other benzodiazepines. Is there another alternative? Levels of neurosteroids have been found to be lower in these patients (Romeo, 1996). The researchers say, "A decrease of neuroactive steroid biosynthesis may contribute to withdrawal symptoms. One can infer that a pharmacologically induced increase of neurosteroid content should be beneficial in the treatment of the withdrawal symptoms in alcoholic subjects."

There have been no formal studies as to whether Preg can be beneficial in decreasing food addiction.

Weight loss

Having experimented with varying doses of Preg, I have not found this hormone to have a significant influence on appetite. Preg is not an appetite suppressant, except perhaps in very high doses. Therefore, most people would likely consume their normal food intake while on low doses of this hormone. However, if Preg improves mood, perhaps some people could lose weight. Overeating (overuse of a substance, such as food) has many causes, including boredom, easy availability of snacks, and as a way to elevate mood. Since Preg provides a wonderful sense of well-being, many users may not feel the need to overindulge in snacks.

In this chapter, and throughout the book, we've seen how Preg can help people improve their lives in a number of areas. In the next chapter, I'll give dosage recommendations to the extent possible based on current research.

CHAPTER 9

THE RIGHT DOSE

Let's assume you and your medical provider have decided that Preg could potentially be of therapeutic benefit. How do you then determine the appropriate dose?

Compounding pharmacies can make Preg available in any prescribed dose from 2 to 100 mg. They can also make Preg in any form, including regular pills, micronized capsules, sublinguals, and creams. Vitamin companies also sell Preg in a variety of forms and dosages. Some also add Vitamin C, Vitamin E, ginkgo, or other nutrients and herbs to their products. You will also find combinations of Preg with DHEA.

As I've said before, we are just beginning to learn about how Preg works within the body, with its roles in brain health and hormone replacement therapy among the most extensively studied aspects of this hormone. Therefore, I cannot provide recommended dosages for a number of the conditions I have discussed in this book. We simply do not have enough information—yet. However, I can provide recommendations, based upon existing studies, for the following conditions.

What you'll find in your local vitamin or retail store

Pills or *capsules* come in dosages of 10, 15, 25, 30, and 50 mg. When Preg is ingested orally, it is absorbed from the intestines into the portal vein, which takes it to the liver. The liver is the chemical factory of the body, and it makes good sense for it to have first crack at the blood supply from the digestive system. Physicians call this the "first-pass effect." Thereafter, Preg makes its way to the rest of the body.

One of the liver's functions is to metabolize sterols and steroids. Because of this, Preg will first be metabolized by the liver into other active and inactive hormones, and the amount of actual Preg that reaches the general circulation will likely be less than the ingested dose.

A way to minimize liver metabolism of steroids is to use *micronized* preparations. Micronization is a process that creates tiny particles that can be absorbed from the intestines into the lymphatic system (which runs along with the intestinal tract) and then into the bloodstream—mostly bypassing the liver.

Sublingual Preg is another route to minimizing liver metabolism of Preg. Sublingual means that you put the tablet under your tongue and let it dissolve. This allows the Preg to be absorbed from the tiny capillaries of the mouth into general circulation. Note that sublingual forms of certain medicines are better absorbed, and thus provide higher concentrations. Sublingual preparations of vitamins, drugs, and herbal extracts are common. Melatonin also comes sublingually. Other forms of Preg that can be absorbed from the mouth include spray, chewing gum, and liquid.

Some people take a regular capsule that's meant to be swallowed, open it, and place a portion of it under the tongue. The result is similar to taking a sublingual preparation. Preg has no inherent taste, unless it's been flavored with mint, orange, or other flavors.

Ointments and *creams* are available through compounding pharmacies or sold at some stores. It is unclear at this time how much Preg can enter through the skin when applied topically. The cream can be applied to many areas of the body, including the chest, abdomen, arms, thighs, and face. If a company claims that they have a yam extract that the body can convert into Preg, be skeptical. Real Preg must be present in the cream.

The sublingual, spray, gum, liquid, and micronized versions of Preg, as well as the creams and ointments, will generally bypass the liver's first-pass effect. Most users notice a clearer or "purer" feeling since more Preg is in an unaltered form as it goes into the bloodstream and then into the brain. I believe you should try several forms to see which ones you prefer. Whether, in the long run, avoiding the liver's first-pass effect is healthier and leads to more beneficial outcomes is not known at this time. Since we don't know which form is healthier, I would recommend using the form that provides you with the best sense of well-being or the most positive effect on your particular medical condition. You can also alternate between different forms, or even combine them.

Preg is a stable molecule and there are no special precautions required for storage (Henderson, 1950). Keep it in a cool, dark area and it should be just fine.

So little research has been done with Preg in humans that the preferred dosages, and the preferred forms of administration, have yet to be established. The amount of Preg used in studies has ranged from one mg to several hundred mg. Since the research in this area is still new, it is best to start with low doses before considering higher ones. I advise supervision by a health care practitioner before using Preg, particularly if you have a medical condition or are taking other medicines. There haven't been enough studies to know how Preg interacts with other medicines and nutrients.

Keeping the above limitations in mind, I have formulated some guidelines of my own. These are based on my experiences in taking Preg, treating patients, talking with hundreds of users, and in my discussions with clinicians who have used this hormone in their practice.

The right dose for mood elevation

Start with a dose of 10 mg in the morning when you get up. (In you're very sensitive to medicines, start with 5 mg.) You can swallow the pill or capsule with just plain water on an empty stomach or with breakfast. Start with 5 mg for sublingual. Take the Preg on a day where you'll have an opportunity to enjoy it. During the day, take a long walk outside in a garden or park, or through a pleasant neighborhood or town. Other options include strolling through a shopping mall, or visiting galleries, antique shops, or museums. If you stay indoors and are distracted by work or other matters, you may not notice Preg's subtle effects.

• If you notice an effect the very first day—such as mood elevation, energy, alertness, visual enhancement, or a steadiness of mood—and you don't experience difficulty sleeping that evening, then 10 mg is probably the right dose for you. If you don't notice an effect, continue with 10 mg each morning for about a week. There's a small possibility that some sensitive individuals may feel overstimulated on 10 mg. In this case, either skip your dose the next day or take 5 mg.

• If, after a week, you still don't notice an effect, increase the dose to 20 mg and continue on this course for another week. If you eventually notice an effect on 20 mg, and you are sleeping well at night, then this could be right for you.

• If you don't notice an effect at 20 mg, then increase the dose to 30 mg and follow the same recommendations. You can gradually increase the dose by 10 mg each week until you reach the desired effect. Some of my patients did not feel an effect until they reached 60 mg. This is unusual.

- Once you've noticed an effect, you can reduce your next day's dose. The reason I say this is because Preg has a long half-life, and it can, in some people, still be around the next day. Preg may accumulate in our tissues, especially the central nervous system. Therefore, each time you take Preg, you could be building up on your previous dose. Once you have loaded yourself with Preg, and know what the effects are, then you don't need as much.

- Occasionally take "hormone holidays" and stop using it for a few days. I say this just to be cautious, since we don't know the long-term effects of regular Preg use.

- If you get insomnia one night, skip your dose the next day; the following day, take 10 mg less. If you are already on a low dose like 10 mg, then take half. Some people find that they notice an effect even on 2 or 3 mg. Initially, it took 30 mg for me to notice the well-being from Preg, but now I notice the mood elevation on even 5 mg. Once you know what it feels like, you are more attuned to the subtle changes that Preg induces.

As a rule, dosages can always be increased if they are too low or ineffective, and decreased if side effects occur or if they work too well. Until we learn more about Preg, the continuous use of this hormone as an antidepressent should be limited to a period of no more than four months.

The right dose for hormone replacement

The following are some rough guidelines on hormone replacement therapy. Please discuss these with your physician if you're planning to take hormones for more than one month.

I wish to emphasize that these are suggestions only; in no way do I suggest that these dosages are right for everyone. Each of you reading this book has a unique biochemistry. Some of you may not need any of these hormones, while others would benefit from higher doses. Also, your health care provider may have a different opinion, believing that the above recommendations are too low, too high, or perhaps inappropriate for you. Listen to your personal physician—he or she knows your medical condition best. At the same time, though, recommend that your physician learn more about Preg if he or she is not familiar with the clinical uses of this hormone.

Men: age 40 to 50

Melatonin: 0.1 to 0.5 mg once or twice a week, an hour or two before bedtime, especially if you have difficulty sleeping.

Plus one of the following:

Preg: 2 to 10 mg in the morning, frequently taking hormone holidays.

Or

DHEA: 2 to 10 mg in the morning, frequently taking hormone holidays.

Or

A combination of Preg and DHEA totaling 2–15 mg.

Men: age 50 to 65

Melatonin: 0.1 to 1 mg once or twice a week, an hour or so before bedtime, especially if you have difficulty sleeping.

Plus one of the following:

Preg: 2 to 15 mg in the morning, frequently taking hormone holidays.

Or

DHEA: 2 to 15 mg in the morning, frequently taking hormone holidays.

Or

A combination of Preg and DHEA totaling 4–20 mg.

Men: age 65 and older

Melatonin: 0.1 to 1 mg once, twice, or three times per week an hour or so before bedtime, especially if you have difficulty sleeping. You could even consider taking 0.1 to 0.5 mg almost every night for chronic insomnia.

Testosterone: Optional, if DHEA by itself does not provide enough of an androgenic effect.

Plus one of the following:

Preg: 5 to 20 mg in the morning, occasionally taking hormone holidays.

Or

DHEA: 5 to 20 mg in the morning, occasionally taking hormone holidays.

Or

A combination of Preg and DHEA totaling 5–25 mg.

Premenopausal women: age 40 to about 50

Melatonin: 0.1 to 0.5 mg once or twice a week, an hour or two before bedtime, especially if you have difficulty sleeping.

Plus one of the following:

Preg: 2 to 8 mg in the morning, frequently taking hormone holidays.

Or

DHEA: 2 to 8 mg in the morning, frequently taking hormone holidays.

Or

A combination of Preg and DHEA totaling 2–10 mg.

Postmenopausal women, 50 to 65

Melatonin: 0.1 to 1 mg once or twice a week, an hour or so before bedtime, especially if you have difficulty sleeping.

Plus one of the following:

Estrogen: Generally half to two-thirds the dose normally recommended. For instance, in the case of Premarin, 0.3 to 0.5 mg would be adequate, instead of 0.625. However, I recommend natural or plant estrogens instead of the synthetic versions or those collected from horse urine. Estrogen is available by prescription only. I also recommend you consume between one and four ounces of a soy product a day. This could be in the form of tofu, soy milk, or another form. Natural estrogens, such as estrone, estriol, and estradiol, as pills or skin patches, are available from compounding pharmacies.

Progesterone: Since Preg converts into progesterone, the use of Preg makes the need for progesterone less essential. If you do take this hormone, use the natural form in micronized, sublingual, or cream forms. You would need a lower dose of progesterone if you're already on Preg. Progesterone, in the appropriate strength, is available by prescription. Weaker strengths are available over the counter.

Plus one of the following:

Preg: 2 to 15 mg in the morning, occasionally taking hormone holidays.

Or

DHEA: 2 to 15 mg in the morning, occasionally taking hormone holidays.

Or

A combination of Preg and DHEA totaling 4–15 mg.

Women over age 65

Melatonin: 0.1 to 1 mg once, twice or three times a week, an hour or so before bedtime, especially if you have difficulty sleeping. You could even consider taking 0.1 to 0.5 mg almost every night if you have chronic insomnia.

Estrogen: See estrogen recommendations on page 88.

Progesterone: See progesterone recommendations on page 88.

Plus one of the following:

Preg: 5 to 15 mg in the morning, occasionally taking hormone holidays.

Or

DHEA: 5 to 15 mg in the morning, occasionally taking hormone holidays.

Or

A combination of Preg and DHEA totaling 5–20 mg.

Some individuals prefer taking a high dose of Preg one day and skipping a dose the next day. If this works well for you, fine. I generally prefer a smaller dose used daily as opposed to disturbing the body's balance with excessive amounts. Dr. Flood agrees: "In general most medicines, except perhaps antibiotics [and certain chemotherapeutic/chronobiotic agents], are better taken to produce steady state levels instead of peaks and troughs. He adds, Practically, this would mean taking a smaller amount of Preg daily rather than a high dose one day and none the next."

Suggested dosages for other conditions

For the treatment of difficult chronic conditions, such as rheumatoid arthritis, the usual effective dose of Preg used in experiments has been 100 to 200 mg. These dosages should definitely *not* be taken without adequate physician supervision, and even then, should be used only a few weeks or less.

It would certainly be worthwhile to give Alzheimer's disease patients 5 to 20 mg of Preg daily. This could be done in as an adjunct to other therapies.

A low dose of Preg, ranging from 5 to 20 mg, should be tried in multiple sclerosis patients under the guidance of a physician.

Preg has not been officially tested in Parkinson's disease, but is certainly worth a try for improvement of overall mental function at a dose of 5 to 20 mg.

I would recommend that anyone who has a problem with arrhythmias, congestive heart failure, or other cardiac abnormalities to start Preg, DHEA, and other hormones in low doses. For instance, open a capsule and start with 2 or 5 mg of Preg. I have heard of anecdotal reports of individuals experiencing episodes of heart irregularities when they took high doses, such as 50 or 100 mg, of Preg or DHEA.

The importance of starting low

My philosophy in using medicines is to start low and gradually increase the dose, thus minimizing or avoiding side effects. Other doctors feel comfortable starting with much higher doses. It's a matter of style and judgment. Over my many years of practicing medicine, I have become much more cautious about dosages. As physicians and individuals, we often blindly follow the package information provided by the drug or vitamin companies, not appreciating the fact that each person is unique. Some people are very sensitive to even minute amounts of medicines.

I also believe in synergism, that is, the use of low doses of many medicines or the combination of a medicine with a natural therapy. For instance, instead of taking a high dose of Preg, such as 50 or 100 mg, for mood elevation, I prefer that someone take 5 or 10 mg but, in addition, incorporate cognitive and behavioral changes. These include reducing stress, taking exercise classes, getting involved in activities with people, finding a passionate goal in life, traveling to exotic places, practicing yoga, and engaging in other enjoyable activities.

As for the long-term use of Preg, the maximum daily dose I recommend at this time is 20 mg. Future studies will tell us whether higher doses for longer periods can be used safely.

Doctors and patients are often looking for the magic pill that, by itself, will cure all ills. The human body is too complicated, with too many biochemical reactions occurring every second, for one pill to be the answer to all problems. The answer lies in intelligently combining a variety of modalities, that is, both pill and non-pill approaches.

Some people call themselves purists and object to the use of medicines, claiming that psychotherapy, along with cognitive or behavioral therapies, are adequate in elevating mood or treating depression. By shunning the intelligent use of these effective hormones, I believe they are short-changing themselves of exceptional therapeutic options.

How soon will I notice an effect from Preg?

Few users who start with 10 mg will feel an effect that very day. When the dose is raised to 20 mg, more will notice a calm, peaceful feeling, often with a sense of heightened alertness and awareness; everything seems more special. Some describe it as being more in touch with one's environment. This becomes even more pronounced when the dose is raised to 30 mg or higher. However, rare individuals will not feel an effect even at 60 mg or higher doses.

Interestingly, once you notice an effect from Preg, you are able to recognize similar effects on following days from much smaller doses. Perhaps Preg accumulates in the brain, or maybe some receptors are sensitized, or the levels of brain chemicals are elevated. We don't yet know the exact reasons.

You should be patient with Preg since, if you're taking a low dose, it sometimes takes two weeks or more to notice the subtle changes. Preg's influence can sometimes be additive, carrying over into subsequent days. On taking a high dose, however, some people may feel more alert and aware relatively fast, even within a half an hour.

Personally, I now notice a clarity in vision, calmness, and mood elevation within one hour of taking 10 mg of Preg, sometimes even sooner. This feeling remains steady most of the day and can last late into the night. Often, music even sounds better.

What time of day should I take Preg?

I recommend that you take it first thing in the morning before or with breakfast, since taking Preg later in the day can lead to excessive alertness and insomnia.

Some people claim that an evening dose works well for them. But since Preg does cause users to be more alert, my concern with evening timing is that it could cause shallow or restless sleep. Then again, some people can drink coffee at night and still sleep well. Each person is unique. Experiment to see whether morning, midday, or evening works better for you.

If you normally get sleepy in the evening and find that 10 mg of Preg in the morning is not enough to keep you alert later in the day, you can split your dose and take the second half before lunch.

Are Preg pills well absorbed?

When you take a Preg pill, it is sulfated in the intestinal system (the mineral sulfur and four oxygen molecules are added) and rapidly absorbed. Thus, Preg-S (or Preg-sulfate) is how this hormone largely circulates in the bloodstream.

Preg is very well absorbed from the intestinal system. In one small study involving three volunteers, 175 mg of Preg was given before a meal and there was a rapid rise—within 1 to 4 hours—in Preg and Preg-S blood levels. After 24 hours, the level of Preg in the blood had returned to normal, but that of Preg-S was still much higher than normal. This indicates that a high dose of Preg can elevate blood levels of Preg-S for quite a long time. This could account for the overstimulation and insomnia felt by people who take large doses.

I'm already on DHEA, can I add Preg?

Whenever you experiment with any medicine or hormone that provides a noticeable feeling, it is best you learn its full effects alone rather than adding it to an existing regimen of medicines and hormones. Therefore, if you already are on DHEA, and you want to add Preg, I recommend you temporarily go off the DHEA. After a few days of being off DHEA, start Preg in the dosage recommendations listed earlier in this chapter.

Once you are fully familiar with the various dosages and forms of Preg, and its multiple effects on your mind and body, then you can re-introduce DHEA in small doses. Remember that both Preg and DHEA have some effects that are similar and their combination would be additive. Therefore, if you already are on 20 mg of Preg, and you add DHEA, the combined dosage should not greatly exceed 20 mg.

Is it okay if I self-medicate with Preg?

Your health care provider should be consulted any time you plan to use hormone supplements regularly. After all, in addition to being converted to progesterone, DHEA and other hormones, Preg has, by itself, multiple influences on the human body. Taking Preg is not as simple as popping a Vitamin C pill.

If your health care provider is not familiar with Preg, lend or give him or her a copy of this book, or other material that provides a well-balanced opinion.

Would testing help you determine your appropriate Preg dosage? We'll explore this issue in the next chapter.

CHAPTER 10

THE PROS AND CONS OF LAB TESTING

After I wrote *DHEA: A Practical Guide,* one of the most common questions I was asked by both DHEA users and doctors who prescribe it concerned the necessity of having laboratory tests done. There are obvious benefits in knowing our hormone levels before supplementing with them for prolonged periods. However, there are also limits to these tests. And would you believe there could be drawbacks?

Normal levels

Blood and saliva levels of Preg and DHEA throughout life have not been thoroughly studied, and you will find different ranges from different laboratories (see table on page 96). Your doctor can order blood levels of Preg, Preg-Sulfate (Preg-S), or 17-hydroxy-Preg. Before Preg gets converted to DHEA, the intermediary hormone is 17-hydroxy-Preg. At this point we don't know for sure which hormone is the preferred one to test and monitor, although it is likely that Preg-S would be a good choice since it is found in much higher concentrations in blood than the other two substances. Saliva Preg levels can also be measured, but there is so little information on this that I do not recommend you exclusively rely on saliva testing at this time.

Blood Levels of Preg

	Preg[1]	Preg-S[2]	17-OH-Preg[3]
Neonates	150–2000 ng[4]/ 100 ml	22–86 mcg[5]/ 100 ml	—
Children	20–140 ng/ 100 ml	—	—
Teenagers	10–150 ng/ 100 ml	—	—
Adults	20–150 ng/ 100 ml	2.7–8 mcg/ 100 ml	30–420 ng/ 100 ml
Postmenopausal Women[6]	5–100 ng/ 100 ml	—	—

1. Preg ranges are from Specialty Laboratories in Santa Monica, California.

2. Preg-S ranges are from *Clinical Guide to Laboratory Tests*, second edition, Norbert Tietz, editor (W.B. Saunders Company, 1990).

3. 17-OH-Preg range is from Corning Laboratories in San Juan Capistrano, California.

4. One gram = 1,000 milligrams (mg) = 1,000,000 micrograms (mcg) = 1,000,000,000 nanograms (ng). One liter equals 1,000 milliliters (ml).

5. Please note that Preg-S levels are in micrograms (mcg). Preg-S levels are 10 to 50 times higher in blood than Preg levels.

6. Postmenopause range provided by Dan Collins, N.D., National Biotech Lab, Seattle, Washington.

Benefits of testing

If you're planning to take Preg for a short period of time for some of the conditions discussed in this book, such as mood elevation, you need not be tested. However, testing becomes a good option when high dosages are being used or when Preg is being considered for long-term hormone replacement therapy.

By knowing your initial levels of Preg, progesterone, DHEA, testosterone, and estrogens, you can better determine which hormones you are deficient in. Through testing you may also find that your levels are quite adequate and you really don't need any of these hormones—yet.

If your levels of these hormones are low, your doctor can recommend an appropriate starting dose. Then, your levels could be monitored in a month or two to see how well you are absorbing these hormone supplements, and how well you are converting them into their metabolites. This can give you and your doctor a better handle on how much to increase or decrease your dosages. If the lab findings show that you're not converting Preg into DHEA, then your physician would recommend adding DHEA to your hormone cocktail.

But is it really this simple?

Limitations of testing

Although levels of Preg can be measured in blood, the research in the field of Preg testing is still new, and few studies have been done to accurately determine the normal levels in different age groups.

Even if we eventually accurately determine the levels of Preg in blood or saliva, this does not tell us the levels of Preg where they really count—that is, within our cells. As Preg-S travels around the bloodstream, it enters organs, tissues, and cells, where it has multiple influences. It is then further metabolized into various other steroid hormones. The conversion of Preg to progesterone, DHEA, and other hormones varies among different tissues and organs. For instance, prostate cells may metabolize Preg differently than ovarian cells, immune cells, or brain cells.

To complicate matters further, the ability of each organ, tissue, or cell to use and metabolize Preg can vary with the time of day and month (especially in premenopausal women). Each person will have a different ability to metabolize and convert Preg into various hormones. Medicines, nutrients, age, and medical conditions can also affect actual Preg levels.

Realizing these limitations, some physicians are not eager to recommend that their patients get expensive tests, especially if Preg is going to be used temporarily for a specific condition or if the dosages used as hormone replacement therapy are low. Other physicians, and patients, feel more comfortable knowing what the levels are, even with the above limitations in mind.

Other factors we need to consider before undergoing expensive testing:

• The type of food we eat can lower or elevate levels of hormones in the blood, thus giving a false reading. For instance, swallowing an estrogen pill with grapefruit juice alters its bioavailability. There are undoubtedly many other food components that interact with steroid hormones.

• When testing for Preg levels, should we also measure levels of its metabolites, such as progesterone, aldosterone, cortisol, DHEA, androstenedione, testosterone, and estrogens? It would make a lot of sense to know how much of the Preg is going into the progesterone pathway and how much is going into the DHEA pathway.

- What about other hormones that theoretically could be influenced by Preg, such as ACTH (adrenocorticotropic hormone), FSH (follicle stimulating hormone), LH (leutenizing hormone), and GH (growth hormone)? And what about dozens of other hormones such as CRH (corticotropin releasing hormone), prolactin, thyroxine, vasopressin, parathyroid, insulin, and others? At what point do we stop measuring all the possible hormones, immune cells, blood lipids, proteins, neurotransmitters, and the myriad other compounds and molecules that circulate in the blood or are present in tissues?

- Could getting the levels of a few hormones give us a false sense of security? Might we think that we know what's going on in our bodies, whereas we could be completely wrong? Preg could accumulate in tissues, especially in the brain and other neural tissues. In one study on human cadavers, it was estimated that the concentration of Preg was more than 70 times higher in the brain than in the blood (Baulieu, 1996). The concentration of DHEA in brain was found to be only six times higher. With continued ingestion of Preg, more and more could accumulate in the brain, while blood levels could remain relatively low. Thus, a physician ordering a blood test could find relatively low levels and be fooled into recommending higher daily doses of Preg, when the patient's brain and other tissues are becoming over-saturated with the hormone.

- Preg could predominantly be metabolized in the progesterone pathway in one tissue or organ, whereas it could predominantly be metabolized to DHEA and the sex steroid pathway in another tissue or organ. Blood levels would only show the combined mix.

- Let's say an older person is tested for levels of Preg or

DHEA and the DHEA level comes back as 100 microgram per 100 ml. The normal ranges in youth is between 200 and 600 mcg/100 ml. How do we know whether this person had a level of 200 in their youth or had a level of 600? If they had a level of 200, and we give this person a lot of DHEA to raise the levels to about 400—the median amount found in young adults—could we be giving this patient excessive doses that could prove counterproductive?

- Thus far we've assumed that the numbers we get back from labs are accurate. But this isn't always the case. Labs make mistakes, too. Since testing for Preg levels is still in its infancy, different labs have different standards and methods. Chris Heward, Ph.D., an endocrinologist from Carlsbad, California, has spent countless hours in laboratories. He tells me, "People believe the results of lab tests as gospel. They don't realize that a number of variables can change the final result. These include the skill of the technician doing the testing, the type of antibody used in the radioimmuno assay test, the freshness of the sample, the time of day or month a sample was taken from the patient, and the calibration of the machine doing the testing."

- I have spoken with directors of different labs regarding saliva testing for DHEA. One director told me that testing DHEAS is preferable to DHEA testing while another director told me the opposite—that DHEAS is actually a contaminant and DHEA testing in saliva is the way to go. Whose opinion can we trust?

- What about the cost of testing? Although simple Preg levels or DHEA levels may not be too expensive to determine, if such tests are repeated several times a year they could add up to thousands of dollars. If the levels of many other hormones are also tested, then the cost could rise astronomically.

● Millions of Americans are using hormone supplements. If everybody who is taking Preg, or DHEA, had thousands of dollars of testing done a year, our health care financing system would go into a crisis. Insurance rates would have to rise dramatically.

Having considered the above benefits and limitations of testing, it will ultimately be up to you, in consultation with your health care provider, to decide whether testing is appropriate. One caution I have is to make sure your physician does not have a financial interest in the laboratory where you are being tested. This could taint his or her recommendation.

One of my patients, age 46, had a low level of DHEA sulfate. When I started her on 5 mg a day, she developed a few pimples. A repeat lab test showed her level to still be low. Thus, according to the lab study, she required more DHEA. However, according to her skin, even 5 mg was too much. Which is more important, the patient or the lab test? *The way a hormone makes you feel, the symptoms you experience, and the influence it has on your tissues, are more important than laboratory test numbers.*

Let's also keep in mind that when doctors prescribe estrogens for women, they rarely check blood levels. They generally just give a standard dose of 0.625 mg, or a predetermined dose on a patch, no matter the age or weight of the patient. Therefore, there is a precedent in medicine of giving hormone replacement without measuring levels.

A better alternative?

As medicine becomes more high tech, doctors often diagnose patients based on results of lab studies rather than through observation skills. In fact, modern physicians have not developed some of the clinical evaluation skills that doctors from previous generations had refined. Instead of a complete evaluation of skin, hair, eyes, weight, muscle tissue, and so on, we often take a short cut and order a battery of tests. I'm sometimes guilty of this, too.

When doctors recommend patients go on hormone replacement, they do so because of the anticipated positive effects on a variety of body organs and tissues. Therefore, why not focus and evaluate these organs and tissues in deciding the appropriate doses of hormones, instead of depending on what the blood, saliva, or urine hormone levels say?

The following are some parameters that should be considered while monitoring someone on hormone replacement therapy. Both the individual taking the hormones and the health care practitioner need to be involved. These are just guidelines. You may consider having less or more done depending on your particular circumstance. Having evaluated tens of thousands of patients over the years, I have realized that some patients want the least done while others want to have every test possible performed. Remember that steroid hormones influence, or are metabolized in, a variety of body tissues, including the liver, fat cells, skin, endometrium, myometrium, intestines, breast, kidney, lung, muscle, heart, brain, prostate, testes, ovaries, eyes, and others.

Here are some general guidelines:

The basics (strongly recommended)
Weight
Blood pressure
Heart rate and rhythm
Muscle mass
Body fat
Eyes
Hearing
Skin, particularly for hair growth, moisture, and
    pimples
Hair

Brain function, such as mood, alertness, memory, motivation
Sleep patterns
Flexibility of joints
Aerobic capacity

Additionally in men
Prostate gland, mostly through finger exam

Additionally in women
Breast tissue, mostly through palpation, and also possibly through mammograms
Uterus and cervix, mostly through Pap tests
Vaginal tissue

Lab tests
Routine blood panel that includes blood count, white count, kidney function, blood sugar, triglycerides, cholesterol, liver enzymes, and thyroid tests
Urinalysis

Other tests that could be done include EKG, chest x-ray, bone densinometry, colonoscope, and PSA (prostate-specific antigen).

My own opinion is that people using Preg for long periods should only be taking low dosages, such as 2 to 15 mg. On these low dosages, regular laboratory testing would not be as essential; testing once a year may be all that's needed.

I urge clinicians to pay more attention to how patients respond to these hormones and how they appear clinically, rather than blindly ordering lots of expensive tests.

Dr. Morley agrees with me. He says:

If someone is on Preg, instead of measuring progesterone, DHEA, sex steroids, and a bunch of hormone levels, I would instead recommend following an individual clinically and also monitoring routine blood studies such as blood count, white count, liver enzymes, and the other routine laboratory tests done during regular checkups. These routine blood studies and the clinical evaluation can give us a better indication of what's going on in the body than just measuring hormone levels.

In the next chapter, I will explain some of Preg's possible side effects, including those that can result from Preg's interactions with medicines and other substances.

CHAPTER 11

CAUTIONS, SIDE EFFECTS, AND DRUG INTERACTIONS

P reg has not been studied as thoroughly as melatonin and DHEA, the two other hormones now sold over the counter. Consequently, we're still in the early stages of learning about this important hormone and its full effects on the human body.

It is best to proceed with caution until more information is available. This means using the lowest effective dosages and seeking supervision by a knowledgeable health care provider. There are many medical or psychiatric conditions in which Preg can be used temporarily and then stopped. With this conservative approach, it is unlikely that any problems would arise. Our major uncertainty at this time involves the long-term use of Preg as hormone replacement therapy, especially if high doses are used.

With time, as more and more people use this hormone, we'll have a fuller understanding of its benefits and side effects. Those who have already found Preg to be helpful in terms of mood elevation, stress reduction, arthritis help, and so forth, but are concerned about unknown long-term effects, may feel more comfortable using Preg only as needed and occasionally taking time off from it. If symptoms recur, they can go back on the hormone. Taking these "hormone holidays" will mitigate any potential unknown risks (they would also reduce any potential unknown benefits).

High dosages of Preg can result in the following side effects.

Overstimulation and insomnia (or shallow sleep)

In order to minimize these side effects, it is important that you engage in physical activity such as walking or exercising during the day. The excess energy and alertness that Preg provides will thus be put to good use. Otherwise, come bedtime, you may still be too alert, restless, and ready to keep going—like those battery-operated toys in TV commercials that keep marching on and on.

Users sometimes find that they wake up earlier in the morning the following day. This means that the Preg is probably still stimulating your central nervous system.

One of the benefits of Preg (and also one of its shortcomings) is that it induces central nervous system excitability and alertness. Therefore, if too-high dosages are taken, the resulting insomnia, or shallow sleep, can have detrimental effects on our health. After all, deep sleep is one of the most crucial aspects of health and immune system maintenance. I believe overstimulation is one of the major shortcomings of Preg. It will make its therapeutic high-dosage use less practical.

If you do overdo, and find that it's now late at night and you're too alert to be able to sleep, take some melatonin at least an hour before bedtime. Preg would be perfect to take on a day when you expect to be going to a party and staying up very late, such as a Friday or Saturday night, or New Year's Eve.

I also need to mention that many people find that they are alert during the day and yet at bedtime the Preg has worn off and they sleep very deeply.

Irritability, anger, or anxiety

Preg can have a biphasic effect: low dosages can be calming, while high dosages can cause tenseness. Diane, a 35-year-old manager of a vitamin company in San Diego, tells me, "I took a 25 mg Preg pill in the morning and felt extremely irritable all day." I recommended that Diane take only 5 or 10 mg, and only once in a while.

The setting of your day can also influence whether you become irritable or whether you enjoy Preg's energy-boosting effects. For instance, if you're overstimulated on Preg and you happen to be in Venice, walking along the canals and fascinated by the architecture of St. Mark's Square, you'll have a great time. If you're overstimulated and happen to be waiting at a long, slow-moving grocery line, or stuck in an office with a demanding boss giving you orders, you're not going to have a pleasant day. Being physically active while on Preg, especially in an outdoor environment, is very important.

Preg can motivate you to get things done. It can make you think faster and clearer. This can have a negative consequence if your quick thinking and problem-solving abilities, whether at home or in the office, cannot be matched by those around you. You may grow impatient when things aren't getting done at a rapid pace.

Another time to avoid a high dose of Preg is when you anticipate an argument or disagreement with someone. Preg can make you snappy and you may say something in an argumentative tone that you could later regret. Preg is similar to other mood-altering medicines and hormones that can either lead to euphoria or dysphoria depending on your mindset and your setting (environment).

You may also find differences among different forms of Preg. When Preg pills are swallowed, the hormone makes its way to the liver, where some or much of it is metabolized into other steroid hormones. In contrast, micronized, cream, or sublingual forms would provide more Preg and less of its metabolites. This Preg could enter the brain and have a different effect on mood than the metabolites made in the liver. I am only speculating here, and I have no scientific proof of this at this time. Experiment with various forms to see which suit your needs best.

Less frequent side effects noted at higher dosages include headaches and negative mood changes. Elevation of blood pressure, acne, facial hair growth, and irregularities of heart rhythm are rare.

I have had three patients whose back pain from sciatica got temporarily worse when they took Preg. They were already experiencing the nerve pain when they added the hormone. Within a day or two, their pain got worse. I'm not sure if this is a coincidence or whether it was due to Preg enhancing pain sensation. We do know that Preg enhances neural perception, including vision and hearing, so it does make sense that it could also make us more aware of neural pain.

Until we learn more, I would caution you not to take high dosages of Preg while you are experiencing neural pain, including back pain, shingles, neck pain, and carpal tunnel syndrome.

Older individuals, particularly those who are on multiple medicines or have chronic medical conditions, should be careful anytime they add any type of supplement to their regimen, especially hormones. We don't know how Preg influences cardiac function or the function of other organs, especially at high dosages. I suspect doses of 2 to 8 mg will not have any detrimental consequences for individuals in frail health.

When not to use Preg

Although no studies have shown Preg to have serious adverse effects, I would nevertheless like to point out some medical conditions where we need to be very cautious. These include:

● **Pregnancy**—We don't have any human studies evaluating the use of Preg in pregnancy.

● **Unstable medical conditions**—If you suffer from cardiac irregularities, or are on multiple medicines, or have an unstable medical condition, make sure you are closely supervised by your physician.

Preg's interactions with other substances

There are no studies published on the combination of Preg with prescription or nonprescription drugs and nutrients. However, based on what is known about Preg and my knowledge of medicine, I can offer some tentative suggestions. We have no definite answers at this time and I am only providing an educated opinion.

Alcohol

According to one study, drinking alcohol can substantially increase estrogen levels in postmenopausal women taking oral estrogens (Ginsburg, 1996). Moderate alcohol consumption tripled circulating levels of estradiol. The researchers state, "Changes in estradiol were significantly correlated with changes in blood alcohol levels. Significant increases in estradiol were detected within 10 minutes after drinking."

I suspect many steroid hormone levels would be affected similarly when moderate amounts of alcohol are consumed. However, an occasional drink is not likely to have much of a clinical influence.

Personally, I've enjoyed an occasional glass of wine while on Preg and found no adverse effects.

Antidepressants

These include the serotonin reuptake inhibitors, such as Prozac, Paxil, and Zoloft, and the tricyclics, such as Elavil, and newer agents, such as Buspar, Serzone, and Effexor. Since Preg is a mood-enhancing hormone, its use may reduce the dosages required for prescription antidepressants. See Chapter 3 for a fuller discussion.

Estrogen

While giving lectures, or during radio interviews, postmenopausal women who take estrogen often ask me whether they can cut down on estrogen while on Preg or DHEA. It's very difficult to give an accurate answer since we have no studies to rely on. Preg is metabolically far removed from estrogens (see the diagram on page 18). Therefore, I recommend continuing the estrogen replacement at this time, but in a lower dose. See Chapter 4 for details.

Melatonin

No formal studies have been done evaluating the combined use of melatonin and Preg. Anecdotal reports from my patients, using Preg regularly and melatonin occasionally for sleep do not indicate any unfavorable interactions. If you take too much Preg you will need a sleep-inducing agent at night to counteract the alertness.

I have taken Preg in the morning and melatonin in the evening on numerous occasions without problems.

Multivitamins and mineral supplements

There are no theoretical reasons why taking Preg in combination with low or moderate doses of vitamins and minerals would pose any problems.

Thyroid medications

Since Preg can act as a stimulant, those on thyroid hormone supplements who wish to use Preg should start with very low dosages, such as 2 to 5 mg.

There are hundreds of medicines and nutrients that Preg can interact with. I suggest you consult a professional health care provider about the appropriateness of taking any medications in combination.

SUMMARY

I would like to briefly recap some of the most important points that have been made in the previous chapters.

Mood—There is little doubt that many users notice mood improvement. They describe it as a sense of well-being, peacefulness, or even mild euphoria. Not everyone, though, notices the subtle effects of Preg. This hormone promises to have great potential as an antidepressant.

Memory—There are rodent studies and limited human experiments that indicate Preg to have a role in memory.

Stress relief—Preg does help many people handle stress better. One shortcoming is that it can, on certain days, lead to irritability and impatience.

Energy—While taking long hikes in the mountains, I have noticed that Preg provides an energy-boosting, antifatigue factor. Human studies done back in the 1940s have also reported this antifatigue finding. Many Preg users claim that they are still alert and active late into the evening, even after a physically strenuous day.

Vision and hearing—I am 100 percent convinced that Preg provides me with enhanced visual and auditory perception. Colors are brighter and clearer, with greater contrast; shapes are more defined; nature is more beautiful. Visits to galleries, museums, and shopping malls are more enjoyable. It's just a wonderful experience to look at things as if you're seeing them for the first time. Awareness of one's environment is definitely heightened. However, not everyone seems to be attuned to this perception enhancement.

Sex drive—There does not appear to be any major influence on libido, although some people notice a slightly higher urge for intimacy.

PMS—There is growing anecdotal evidence that many women who suffer from premenstrual syndrome are helped by Preg.

Weight loss—No clear answers are available at this time as to Preg's influence on body fat and weight. In most cases, appetite is not greatly changed.

Muscles—Preg is not as anabolic a hormone as is as DHEA. To quickly and safely gain muscle mass, consider the nutrient creatine. See *Creatine: Nature's Muscle Builder*.

Arthritis—Preg, in combination with other nutrients such as glucosamine, can help ease arthritic aches and pains.

Autoimmune disorders—Preg should be considered as an addition to other therapeutic regimens in the fight against these diseases.

Cancer—Hardly anything is known on Preg's influence in tumor inhibition or promotion.

Heart disease—Again, little is known. Those with cardiac irregularities or severe heart failure should start Preg cautiously.

Osteoporosis—Little is known.

Hormone replacement—I believe that Preg, if used appropriately, can have a tremendous influence on the quality of life of a large number of middle-aged and older individuals. It can be used in combination with other hormones.

Antiaging—As to whether regular use of Preg will help us live longer is not clear at this time. My guess is that we'll eventually find Preg does positively influence longevity.

Final commentary

Now that Preg is being sold over the counter, many people will start using it. Soon, we'll have a tremendous number of anecdotes that will vastly increase our knowledge. Then it's only a matter of time until the pieces of the puzzle start to fit together.

Unfortunately, few formal human studies are ongoing at this time, since many scientists involved in the field of steroid hormone research are concentrating their efforts on estrogen, testosterone, progesterone, and DHEA. Therefore, our knowledge about Preg, at least in the near future, will mostly come from individuals using this hormone and the clinical experience of physicians who prescribe Preg for their patients.

If you wish to keep up to date with the latest research on life extension, Preg, melatonin, DHEA, progesterone, creatine, glucosamine, and other hormones and supplements, subscribe to *Longevity Research Update* (see last three pages).

SHOULD PREG BE SOLD WITHOUT A PRESCRIPTION?

In October, 1994, the Dietary Supplement Law was passed by Congress, making it easier for manufacturers and drug/vitamin stores to sell any vitamin, mineral, herb, nutrient, amino acid, food extract, or any derivative of these supplements without FDA approval. As you can see from the diagram on page 18, Preg is a derivative of cholesterol. Cholesterol itself is derived from the foods we eat, such as meats, eggs, poultry, butter, and dairy products. The body, especially the liver, also produces cholesterol. Therefore, even though Preg is a steroid hormone, it is still considered a food derivative, and thus does not appear to fall under the jurisdiction of the FDA. The FDA could pull this steroid hormone off the market if there were reports of serious side effects. At the time of printing of this book, none had been reported.

What is a steroid hormone?

A steroid is any chemical substance with four carbon ring structures attached to each other. Cortisol, DHEA, testosterone, Preg, progesterone, and estrogen are all steroid hormones that chemically look very similar to each other. As you can see from the diagram on page 18, structurally, they differ from each other in only small ways. However, even tiny changes in the chemical makeup of a substance can cause enormous differences in how it functions and what role it plays in the chemical factories of our bodies.

For instance, testosterone, the male hormone, is only slightly different chemically from estrogen, the female hormone. Yet that slight difference causes men to grow facial hair and women to develop breasts.

Many people think of the word steroid as a synthetic substance used by body builders and weight lifters to boost muscle mass. These types of synthetic steroids are called anabolic steroids and do influence muscle growth at the expense of potentially serious side effects. Preg is not considered an anabolic steroid.

Should Preg be sold without a prescription?

There are both potential benefits and unknown consequences when hormones are easily available to the public. When people see a supplement on the shelf of a store, they have the misconception that everything is known about this supplement and that it has been found to be completely safe. Angela, a small, thin, 43-year-old artist whom I recently met on a hike told me, "I saw a woman on TV who claimed DHEA increased her sex drive. I immediately went to the vitamin store and bought a bottle. I've been taking 50 mg of DHEA for the past three months."

"That's way, way too much for your age and size," I replied. "We don't know the consequences of taking high doses of DHEA for a long time. You should drop your dose to 5 mg and see a doctor to be supervised."

"Since it's over-the-counter, doesn't that mean the FDA

has found it to be safe?" she naively responded.

Angela, and many other people, don't know about the 1994 Dietary Supplement Law.

I believe that Preg and DHEA should be available without a prescription, but in no more than 10 mg dosages. I get uneasy when I see ads marketing the higher dosages, especially the 50 and 100 mg. Let's look at some of the potential benefits of Preg, and at some of the possible objections.

Potential benefits:

- The availability of Preg will accelerate public interest in this hormone. This will encourage more researchers to study it and Preg will re-emerge after four decades of obscurity. We may find some exceptional therapeutic potentials for Preg that other medicines can't easily provide.

- The health, mood, and well-being of millions of people could be improved.

- The availability of effective and fascinating over-the-counter supplements will lead a larger segment of the population to learn more about nutrition, medicine, and their bodies. They will take a more active role in their personal health care. This will also accelerate the rate of public interest in a variety of other natural therapies. Doctors, and the medical establishment, will have to listen to the requests and demands of their patients, and eventually incorporate more natural methods of treatment into their practice.

There is already a mini-revolution going on in medicine. This revolution has started from the bottom up. By this I mean that patients are going to their doctors armed with all the new information on supplements they have read about. They are requesting that their doctors, in turn, learn more about natural nutrients and therapies. Many doctors are listening. Our research center frequently gets calls from doctors who want to schedule a consultation, purchase our books, or subscribe to our newsletter, simply because these provide the type of information that they cannot find in standard medical books and journals.

CRITICS WILL CHARGE:

Some people will take too much Preg for too long, producing untoward effects

They have a valid point, especially when high dosages are sold. As with anything available over the counter, some people will misuse it. However, if someone takes too much Preg, they will get overstimulated, have headaches and insomnia. This would induce them to reduce dosage or stop taking it completely. The fact that a few people may misuse Preg should not be used as a reason to prohibit the majority of intelligent users from having access to it.

If our society allows such extremely dangerous substances as alcohol and tobacco to be sold without a prescription, then there is little justification that this same society shouldn't allow Preg, a much safer substance, to also be available. Let's keep in mind that engaging in such sports as football or skiing is significantly more dangerous then supplementing with natural hormones.

Preg is not approved by the FDA and thus is not safe

Vitamin C is not approved by the FDA either. Come to think of it, neither is water. None of the natural supplements are approved by the FDA, nor do they legally need to be.

FDA approval is very helpful, but does not completely safeguard us against potentially dangerous substances being marketed. In January 1997, I got a letter from Abbott

Pharmaceutical Company advising me that Cylert (pemoline), a FDA-approved drug used as a weight loss agent and for children with attention deficit disorder, can cause acute liver failure. The letter says, "Since Cylert's marketing in 1975, 13 cases of acute hepatic failure have been reported to the FDA. This estimate may be conservative because of under reporting and because the long latency between initiation of Cylert treatment and the occurrence of hepatic failure. Of the 13 cases reported as of May 1996, 11 resulted in death or liver transplantation." I wonder how many incidents of mild or moderate liver, and other bodily damage, have occurred from Cylert and other drugs that have never been reported.

Does this mean that we should never use drugs approved by the FDA? Of course not. My reason for mentioning the above example is to counter arguments by critics who insist that the FDA's waving of their magic wand assures a medication is safe. Natural supplements have, generally, proven to have a far, far better safety record than pharmaceutical drugs.

The purity of over-the-counter products cannot be guaranteed

True, but except for a problem with tryptophan contamination that occurred a few years ago, no major cases of contamination have been reported with supplements. Let's also keep in mind that each year thousands of Americans die, and hundreds of thousands become ill, from contaminated food and water. FDA-approved drugs have occasionally also been found to be contaminated.

The accuracy of labeling of over-the-counter products cannot be guaranteed

True, but almost all products made by reliable vitamin companies are generally of good quality. In January 1997, our research center commissioned an independent laboratory to evaluate more than a dozen DHEA products available on the shelves of vitamin and retail stores. We found that all products contained 90% or more of the amount of DHEA promised on the label. Many of the products were 100% accurate. The results were published in the January, 1997 issue of *Longevity Research Update*, and posted at our web site at http://www.raysahelian.com.

Our research center plans to continue spot evaluations of different DHEA and Preg products and post them on our web site. This should motivate manufacturers and distributors to keep on their toes.

Unexpected reactions or side effects may occur

These are unlikely to occur on the low dosages that I recommend.

Long-term effects of chronic use are unknown

True, but I'm generally suggesting that Preg be used occasionally, or if used regularly for long periods of time, I recommend taking hormone holidays. The only major exception would be as hormone replacement therapy for older individuals. Even then, I feel comfortable that low doses of Preg, such as 5 to 10 mg, should not present any significant problems when used under the guidance of a health care practitioner. In fact, it's possible that not taking any hormones as we age could have more risk than judicious supplementation.

PERSONAL STORIES
OF PREG USERS

Science generally frowns on anecdotes, and for good reason: they can sometimes be misleading and even inaccurate. Nevertheless, when no formal, double-blind, placebo-controlled studies are available, anecdotes are our only source of information. When similar experiences are mentioned by a number of unrelated individuals, it becomes harder for a skeptic to casually dismiss this information.

Physicians

Stan Bazilian, M.D., is a psychiatrist in private practice in Philadelphia, Pennsylvania. He has used Preg in his practice and has found it to be helpful in improving memory, energy, and mood. "Some of my patients find that Preg gives them an undefinable youthful feeling they had not experienced for a long time. I believe Preg should be considered as an adjunct to pharmaceutical drugs in the treatment of depression," he says.

Susan Busse, M.D., a family physician in Palatine, Illinois, has treated close to a hundred patients with Preg. She tells me, "I use Preg for those who can't tolerate the androgenic effects of DHEA. Preg makes my patients have more energy. They feel more alert and have a sense of well-being. I've also found it slightly useful in Alzheimer's patients in terms of better cognition but it's hard to ascribe these effects solely to Preg since I also use other supplements, including ginkgo. When the dose of Preg exceeds 30 mg, side effects can occur. "Spaciness" is how one patient described it. I'm also using it in patients for whom I want to increase progesterone levels, such as postmenopausal women, especially if both their DHEA and progesterone levels are low.

Paul Yanick, Ph.D., in Montclair, New Jersey, has coordinated the therapy of over 100 individuals on Preg, usually at a dose of 10 to 40 mg. He finds that Preg improves mental function and memory. "Patients notice a sense of well-being, are more focused, and have clearer thinking," he says.

INDIVIDUALS

Peppy all day . . . and night

My boyfriend told me about Preg. I purchased 25 mg pills in a local health food store and took one at 2 pm. Preg certainly gave me a boost in energy and made me more alert with a heightened sense of awareness. I was extremely energetic and productive, although I didn't sleep well that night and the aftereffects that occurred the next day were somewhat counterproductive. I felt a bit fatigued, had a slight headache, and a general malaise. Ten days later, I took 10 mg in the morning, and this was just right.

Gina, registered nurse, 36, Las Vegas, Nevada

No more mood swings

For the past two months I've taken 10 mg of Preg and feel more energetic. My mood swings are gone. Interestingly, I seem to be more aware of my environment. So far I've recommended Preg to three patients, and one of them reported that Preg had an antidepressant effect.

Julie, 47, psychotherapist, Minneapolis, Minnesota

Preg and DHEA combo

I'm a 45-year-old medical technologist and I've suspected for a long time that there was a problem with my adrenal glands. Perhaps I have a mild case of Addison's disease, since I've always felt chronically weak and had low blood pressure. A number of conditions came up within the last month that prompted me to try anything. My arthritis was getting worse, my hair was falling out more, I couldn't sleep, and I kept drinking coffee all day as an energy booster. I read about DHEA and Preg and decided to give them a try. I started with 25 mg of Preg and 25 mg of DHEA in the morning. The results were profound. All my symptoms disappeared within days. I also noticed a positive effect on my libido.

Arthur, Philadelphia, Pennsylvania

Insomnia

When I was taking 20 mg of Preg I had problems with insomnia. Now I take 10 mg every other day and it works great. I notice a sense of well-being. My mood is stable . . . organic. I also have less fatigue.

Luis, doctor, Corozal, Puerto Rico

Coffee blues gone

I drink coffee a few times a week in the morning to help me keep alert. However, I often get a slight nervousness or low mood after drinking the coffee. Now that I'm on 10 mg of Preg, I don't seem to get these adverse feelings anymore. Preg keeps me in an even mood, and just as alert as drinking coffee.

I've also found that Preg makes me more focused, yet relaxed. I can get more writing done. Even though I'm using Preg often, I don't think it's habit forming since I often forget to take it.

Audrey, 30, Los Angeles, California

Wired

Someone at the health food store told me to start with 50 mg. The next morning I took this dose and half an hour later felt like I was on amphetamines. It was pleasant. I went through the day fine, but at midnight when I went to bed I was wired. I lay in bed tossing and turning and couldn't get a good night's sleep. The next day I felt shaky and tired. I'm going to try 10 mg next time.

DM, 55, Reno, Nevada

Fibroids less, pimples more

I have been on Preg, 25 mg a day, for the past three months and have noticed the following:

- The fibroid tissue in my breast is much less prominent to my touch

- My breasts have not become sore before my periods as would normally happen

- I do not feel as much pressure in my abdomen from uterine fibroids as I used to.

My face was completely clear of acne during my period when I was on 25 mg a day. However, when I increased my dose to 50 mg, I broke out with pimples.

Evangelina, 47, Austin, Texas

Wicked headaches on high dosage

When we first got Preg in our health food store, it came in a 50 mg strength and I started taking two tablets daily. Within four days I had wicked headaches. Now I'm taking 25 mg every other day. I notice clarity in thinking and a nice sense of well-being. Interestingly, I feel calmer—I'm able to handle all the questions posed by the customers without getting irritated. There's been no noticeable change in libido or sleep.

Jesse, 40, nutrition store manager, Santa Barbara, California

Wouldn't want to live without it

Preg is wonderful. I would never want to live without it. Since I've been on it for two months, I feel more vigorous and energetic. My temperament is mellower and more upbeat; I'm not as much of a type A person anymore.

My sexual interest has slightly increased. This may be psychological since I feel better about myself, and more desirable. I would say that even my self-esteem is better.

DS, 57, Greenville, Maine

Fewer aches and pains

I have mild chronic aches and stiffness in my joints. Nothing unusual, just the normal stiffness common in middle age. I first tried Preg at 10 mg and did not notice an effect. I gradually increased my dose to 20 mg over a period of two weeks and realized that my body was not stiff anymore. My joints weren't hurting. I also noticed a good, overall, balanced well-being. The effect of Preg is subtle but noticeable. When I run out of the Preg, I still feel the positive effects for an additional day. Two days after stopping it, I noticed the stiffness come back in my joints. I did not have any side effects while taking Preg except one night of insomnia when I took 30 mg.

Barbara, 53, Marina Del Rey, California

More alert at night

For many years I've been getting sleepy around 10 p.m. I normally need to go to bed at midnight. Often, I end up taking a two- or three-hour nap at 10 p.m. and then waking up at 1 a.m. or so and not being able to fall back asleep. This has led to a vicious cycle of feeling tired during the day and sleepy again before my bedtime.

I started with 10 mg of Preg in the morning, increased it to 20 mg after a few days, and noticed that I was alert in the evening up to bedtime. Preg has been of significant help in this regard. My sleep at night has not been affected.

I'm also on an antidepressant called Wellbutrin at 75 mg at night. Preg does not seem to have interfered with this medicine.

WD, 53, Marina Del Rey, California

Chores are more pleasant

I've been taking 10 to 20 mg of Preg for the past eight months. I now get more pleasure out of doing tasks that previously seemed burdensome. These include filing and a variety of office tasks.

Will, 52, Petaluma, California

Breast tenderness gone

I was about to start my period (I can tell since my breasts get tender) when I took 10 mg of micronized Preg. Within a day, my breast tenderness went away.

Audrey, 31, Hollywood, California

Skin sensation returns

I've been taking many supplements and antioxidants since 1981, and few things have an effect on me. I started Preg at 25 mg twice a day. It seemed to help me recover from nerve damage caused from a 5th lumbar spondy-lolisthesis (forward movement of the body of one of the lower lumbar vertebrae on the vertebra below it). A year ago, I had numbness on my left thigh from the hip down to knee. I believe Preg helped return the sensitivity within one month.

I feel good and haven't had any side effects.

Warren, 58, Greenville, Maine

Conversation is clearer

I was at my office desk having a conversation with a co-work-er when I suddenly realized how clearly I could understand the information he was presenting and how static-free the conversation was proceeding. At the same time, my vision became awesomely clear!

Rezza, Anaheim Hills, California

PMS is relieved

For two months now I've been using 10 mg of Preg every other day for PMS, starting about two weeks before my peri-od. Preg has definitely decreased the abdominal cramping and soreness in my breast. My mood is even and I don't feel as stressed. My husband is very happy and insists on paying for the Preg bottles.

Kelley, Santee, California

Feels like a dancer

Preg make me feel like a dancer and a model. I walk tall and feel like I'm a piece of fluid art walking through time and space.

Natasha, artist, Marina Del Rey, California

Unusual endurance

I took 10 mg for a week and didn't notice anything. Last week, I increased the dose to 20 mg. Yesterday, I noticed that I had unusual endurance. In the morning I washed my car . . . twice, and then waxed it (I hadn't washed it myself for seven years, always taking it to the car wash). Later I cleaned the kitchen floor, went food shopping, washed the windows, put everything around the house in order, cooked dinner, took care of my 5 year old, read stories to her, and at 11 pm I felt like I could still keep going. Normally I'm exhausted by 9 pm.

I think Preg makes me more motivated. Instead of procrastinating, I get things done. I don't know if this has anything to do with Preg, but my skin feels softer.

Shelley, 43, Laguna Hills, California

AN INTERESTING
CASE HISTORY

This clinical history is presented in cooperation with Dr. Karlis Ullis, M.D., a physician in private practice in Santa Monica, California. I am coordinating, with Dr. Ullis, the evaluation of Preg as an antidepressant of mood and as hormone replacement in the clinical setting.

Arthur, an 80-year-old retired dentist, had a history of prostate cancer and subsequently had his testicles removed in 1991. The testicles were surgically removed in order to reduce testosterone production. Excess testosterone is thought to aggravate prostate cancer.

Since his prostate cancer and testicular surgery, Arthur has had progressive memory loss. He consulted Dr. Ullis in June of 1996 to see if anything could be done. Lab studies at the time showed:

- Total testosterone—almost zero

- DHEAS—almost zero

- Total estrogens—36 picograms per ml (normal for his age and sex, 40 to 115)

- Cortisol—13 micrograms per 100 ml (normal 4 to 22)
- Progesterone—levels were not done
- Pregnenolone—levels were not done

Dr. Ullis started Arthur on 5 mg of Preg in the morning, and the dosage was gradually increased to 120 mg over the next few months. A dose of 120 mg is considered excessive. However, Arthur's case was an exception. Since he was extremely deficient, it was felt appropriate to give him a larger dose than normal. DHEA was initially not given since there was a concern of its conversion into testosterone and the theoretical risk of prostate gland cancer activation.

In January 1997, a blood test was done which showed:

- Total testosterone—less than 10 nanograms per 100 ml (normal 270 to 1070 in adults, less in old age)
- DHEAS—went up to 45 micrograms per 100 ml (normal for his age group, 60 to 100)
- Total estrogens—38 picrograms per ml (normal 40 to 115)
- Cortisol—17.3 micrograms per 100 ml (normal 4 to 22)
- Progesterone—1.9 nanograms per ml (normal 0.3 to 1.2)
- Pregnenolone—30 nanograms per 100 ml (normal 20 to 150 in adults, lower as one ages)

As you can see from the above results, Preg supplementation increased DHEA levels, and, we presume, also increased progesterone levels (we don't have a pretreatment progesterone level). Testosterone and estrogen levels were only minimally affected. We can guess, therefore, that in an older individual, conversion of Preg to immediate downstream hormones such as DHEA and progesterone can be done easily, but conversion into further downstream hormones such as testosterone and estrogens may be more difficult. I suspect young people would have less difficulty in converting Preg into androgens and estrogens.

Further laboratory studies on humans will give us a clearer idea on whether most older individuals will find it difficult to convert Preg into androgens and estrogens. If this is confirmed, it adds more credence to the concept of hormone replacement in the very old using small amounts of a variety of different hormones. See Chapter 5 for practical suggestions.

Another interesting observation is that progesterone levels were high while on Preg. This could mean that Preg replacement may make the need for progesterone less crucial.

Since the start of therapy with Preg, Arthur's memory has stabilized and there has been no further deterioration. His dose of Preg has been reduced to 60 mg and a small amount of DHEA, 10 mg, is being cautiously added to see if it can provide Arthur with additional clinical benefits.

GLOSSARY

Acetylcholine—a chemical found in the nervous system and used to transmit nerve impulses. In the brain, acetylcholine is involved with memory.

ACTH (adrenocorticotrophic hormone)—a hormone secreted by the pituitary gland. It stimulates the adrenal gland to make steroids.

Aldosterone—a steroid hormone produced by the adrenal cortex. Its major function is to facilitate potassium exchange for sodium in the kidney, causing sodium reabsorption and potassium excretion. This leads to the raising of blood pressure. Aldosterone is thus involved in telling our kidneys to maintain high amounts of sodium within our blood so that our blood pressure doesn't fall. When our diet has too little sodium, more aldosterone is released. When we consume a lot of sodium, such as from table salt or potato chips, very little aldosterone is made. Western societies have much sodium in their diet, and thus Americans and Europeans make low amounts of aldosterone.

Alzheimer's disease—a progressive brain disease leading

to memory loss, interference with thinking abilities, and other losses of mental powers. Brain cells show degenerative damage.

Amino acid—a molecule that serves as a unit of structure of proteins and contains nitrogen. Twenty-two amino acids are found in the human body, such as arginine, lysine, tryptophan, and phenylalanine. Eight out of the twenty-two are essential, that is, the body cannot make them. They need to be ingested through foods.

Androgen—a hormone that encourages the development of male sexual characteristics. Some of the androgens made by the adrenal glands are DHEA, DHEAS, androstenedione, and testosterone.

Antibody—a protein produced in response to contact of the body with an antigen. It has the specific capacity of neutralizing an antigen.

Antigen—a substance, bacteria, virus, or toxin to which the body reacts by forming antibodies.

Antioxidant—a substance that combines with damaging molecules and neutralizes them, and thus prevents the deterioration of DNA, RNA, lipids, and proteins. Vitamins C, E, and beta-carotene are the best known antioxidants, but more and more are being discovered each year. It is believed that one aspect of aging is the slow degeneration and breakdown of chemicals within our cells. Antioxidants are thought to prevent or slow down this degenerative process. Melatonin is an antioxidant.

Autoimmune—immunity against self. The body makes antibodies that attack and damage its own cells. Systemic lupus erythematosus is one such condition.

Benzodiazepine—a class of medicines such as Valium,

Dalmane, and Restoril that act on GABA receptors to induce relaxation and sleep. Too much, used too often, can lead to memory loss.

Cell membrane—a thin layer consisting mostly of fatty acids that surrounds each cell.

Cholesterol—the most abundant steroid in animal tissues. It is present in some of the foods we eat. Our liver can also make some if there's not enough in our diet.

Control—in any study, whenever a group of animals or humans are given a certain medicine, they are compared with another group of animals or humans who are in under the same circumstances for everything except the medicine. This second group is known as the controls. This way, researchers can find out what the role of the medicine was independent of any other factors.

Cortisol—a sterol (related to steroid) secreted by the human adrenal glands. High doses lead to interference with the proper functioning of the immune system.

Cytomegalovirus—a type of virus that can invade cells of many organs, but especially the salivary glands. A person with a normal immunity generally would not succumb to this virus.

Diosgenin—a sapogenin derived from the saponins discin and trillin, which are found in the roots of plants such as the yam. In the laboratory, parts of this molecule can be cleaved in order to make certain steroids. The steroid portion, 5-spirostene, serves as a source from which pregnenolone and progesterone can be prepared. Our bodies are not known to have the proper enzymes to convert diosgenin into pregnenolone, progesterone or DHEA. Therefore, ingesting wild yam extracts will not lead to DHEA production.

Epinephrine—a hormone made by the medulla of the adrenal gland and also made in the brain and other parts of the nervous system. The product name is Adrenalin. It is a potent stimulator of heart rate, tightens some blood vessels and relaxes others, and relaxes the bronchi (tubes) in the lungs. In the brain it is considered a neurotransmitter that leads to alertness and vigilance. Epinephrine is made by the amino acids phenylalanine and tyrosine.

Estrogen—a hormone made by the ovaries, adrenal glands, and also in various cells of the body. Estrogen promotes female characteristics. The most common estrogens are estrone, estradiol, and estriol. Premarin, the product name of conjugated estrogens, is actually derived from the urine of horses.

GABA—gamma amino butyric acid, a brain chemical that causes sedation. Medicines such as Valium act on receptors for GABA to induce relaxation.

Glucocorticoid—any steroid-like compound capable of significantly influencing some aspects of metabolism, such as the promotion of glycogen deposition in the liver, and having anti-inflammatory effects. Cortisol is the most potent of the naturally occurring glucocorticoids, but some synthetic derivatives, such as prednisone, are more potent.

Glutamate— an amino acid found in proteins that also acts as a neurotransmitter in the brain.

Gonad—a testicle or ovary.

Hormone—a chemical messenger produced by a gland or organ that influences a number of metabolic actions in our cells. Some hormones have been studied for a number of years, such as estrogen, which has been given to women after menopause for over 20 years.

Hypothalamus—a small area of the brain above and behind the roof of the mouth. The hypothalamus is prominently involved with the functions of the autonomic nervous system and the hormonal system. It also plays a role in mood and motivation.

Immune globulins—a group of proteins found in blood. Immune globulins (or immunoglobulins) fight off infections by attaching to and killing bacteria and viruses. The best known is gamma globulin.

Insulin—a hormone made by the pancreas that helps regulate blood sugar levels.

Interferon—a small protein produced by white blood cells to fight infections, especially viral, and some forms of cancer.

Interleukin—similar to interferon, a small protein produced by white blood cells to fight infections and some forms of cancer. There are many types of interleukins, numbered 1, 2, 3, up to 10 or more. Some interleukins are good, others may have negative effects.

Libido—sex drive.

Lymphocyte—a type of white blood cell. Two major types are B lymphocytes and T lymphocytes.

Lymphokine—a substance released by lymphocytes to help with the immune function. Interferon is a type of lymphokine.

Lymphoma—any of a group of diseases characterized by painless, progressive enlargement of lymph glands. Hodgkin's disease is a form of lymphoma.

Macrophage—a large cell of the immune system that has the ability to be phagocytic, that is, to engulf and kill germs.

This cell is also thought to be involved in plaque formation in arteries.

Metabolism—the chemical and physical processes continuously going in the body involving the creation and breakdown of molecules.

Molecule—the smallest possible quantity of atoms that retains the chemical properties of the substance. For instance, the molecules of water consist of three atoms—two are hydrogen, and one is oxygen.

Multiple sclerosis—a chronic disease in which there is loss of myelin (the covering of a nerve) of the central nervous system. It is characterized by speech defects and loss of muscular coordination.

Mycobacteria—mycobacterium is the singular; a type of bacterium within the same genus as the ones that cause tuberculosis and leprosy. It has the shape of a rod and is gram positive.

Natural killer cell—a type of white blood cell that can destroy certain cancer cells and germs.

Neuron—a brain cell. There are over 100 billion of these cells in our brain. Neurons communicate with each other through chemicals called neurotransmitters.

Neurotransmitter—a biochemical substance, such as norepinephrine, serotonin, dopamine, phenylethylamine, acetylcholine, and endorphin, that relays messages from one neuron to another.

NMDA—not to be confused with the popular street drug MDMA, a.k.a. "Ecstasy"; a type of receptor on our neurons (brain cells). It stands for N-methyl-D-aspartate. This receptor plays an important role in regulating the function and form of synapses on our neurons, thus influencing learning and memory. Aging is thought to be associated with a decline in the number of NMDA receptors, which may partly account for loss of learning ability and memory in old age. Interestingly, the administration of acetyl-l-carnitine (a nutrient, and antioxidant, found in vitamin stores) slows the age-associated reduction in the number of these receptors in rodents (Castorina, 1993.)

Norepinephrine—a hormone made by the adrenal medulla. It is similar in some ways to epinephrine but weaker.

Placebo—a dummy pill that contains no active ingredient.

Platelet—a small, round or oval cell found in the blood involved in blood clotting.

Precursor—a substance that precedes, and is the source, of another substance.

Prostate gland—a partly muscular gland surrounding the urethra at the base of the bladder. It secretes a lubricating fluid that is discharged with the sperm. Enlargement of this gland is known as BPH, benign prostatic hypertrophy.

Receptor—a special arrangement on a cell that recognizes a molecule and interacts with it. This allows the molecule to either enter the cell or stimulate it in a specific way.

Sebaceous gland—a gland in the skin that usually opens into the hair follicles and secretes an oily, semifluid substance known as sebum.

Serotonin—a brain chemical (neurotransmitter) that relays messages between brain cells (neurons). It is one of the primary mood neurotransmitters. It is derived form the amino acid tryptophan. Serotonin can also be converted to melatonin.

Sterol—a steroid of 27 or more carbon atoms with one OH (alcohol) group. Cholesterol is a sterol.

Testosterone—a hormone made by the testicles and adrenal glands, and also in various cells of the body, that promotes masculine traits.

Triglyceride—a type of fat that circulates in the bloodstream. A glycerol molecule forms the backbone to which one, two, or three fatty acids attach. High blood triglyceride levels can lead to atherosclerosis (blockage of arteries).

REFERENCES

Akwa Y, Young J, Kabbadj K, Sancho M, Zucman D. *Neurosteroids: biosynthesis, metabolism and function of pregnenolone and dehydroepiandrosterone in the brain.* J Steroid Biochem Mol Biol 40: 71–81, 1991.

Angeli A, Dogliotti L, Naldoni C, et al. *Steroid biochemistry and categorization of breast cyst fluid: relation to breast cancer risk.* J Steroid Biochem Mol Biol 49:333–39, 1994.

Araghiniknam M, Chung S, Nelson-White T, Eskelson C, Watson R. *Antioxidant activity of dioscorea and DHEA in older humans.* Life Sci 59:PL147–57, 1996.

Barbaccia ML, Roscetti G, Trabucchi M, et al. *Neurosteroids in the brain of handling-habituated and naive rats: effect of CO2 inhalation.* Eur J Pharmacol 261:317–20, 1994.

Baulieu EE, Robel P. *DHEA and DHEAS as neuroactive neurosteroids.* J of Endocrinol 150: S221-S239, 1996.

Belluzzi A. N Eng J Med 334:1557–60, 1996.

Brod S, Lindsey W, Wolinsky J. *Multiple Sclerosis: Clinical*

143

presentation, diagnosis and treatment. American Family Physician 54:1301–11, 1996.

Castorina M, et al. *A cluster analysis study of acetyl-l-carnitine effect on NMDA receptors in aging.* Experimental Gerontology 28:537–48, 1993.

Cavallo MG. Lancet 348:926–28, 1996.

Davis S, Burger H. *Androgens and the Postmenopausal Woman.* J Clin Endocrinol Metab. 81:2759–63, 1996.

Davison R, Koets P, Kuzell W. *Excretion of 17-ketosteroids in ankylosing spondylarthritis: a preliminary report.* J Clin Endocrinol 7:201–04, 1947.

Dennerstein L, Spencer-Gardner C, Gotts G. *Progesterone and the premenstrual syndrome: a double blind crossover trial.* British Med J 290:1617–21, 1985

Flood J, Farr S, Kaiser F, La Regina M, Morley F. *Age-related decrease of plasma testosterone in SAMP8 mice: replacement improves age-related impairment of learning and memory.* Physiol Behav 57(4): 669–73, 1995. Immediate post-training, stereotactically guided, intraparenchymal administration of Preg in the amygdala, septum, mammillary bodies, or caudate nucleus and of Preg-S, DHEAS and corticosterone into the hippocampus was performed in mice weakly trained in a foot-shock active avoidance paradigm. "The finding that fewer that 150 molecules of Preg-S significantly enhanced post-training memory processes when injected into the amygdala establishes Preg-S as the most potent memory enhancer yet reported and the amygdala as the most sensitive brain region for memory enhancement by any substance yet tested."

Flood J, Morley J, Roberts E. *Memory-enhancing effects in male mice of pregnenolone and steroids metabolically derived from it.* Proc Natl Acad Sci USA 89:1567–71, 1992.

Flood J, Morley J, Roberts E. *Pregnenolone sulfate enhances post-training memory processes when injected in very low doses into limbic system structures: the amygdala is by far the most sensitive.* Proc Natl Acad Sci USA 7;92:10806–10, 1995.

Freeman H, Pincus G, et al. *Oral steroid medication in rheumatoid arthritis.* J Clin End 10:1523–32, 1950.

George M, Guidotti A, Rubinow D, Pan B, Mikalauskas K, Post R. *CSF neuroactive steroids in affective disorders: pregnenolone, progesterone, and DBI.* Biological Psychiatry 35 (10): 775–80, 1994.

Ginsburg E et al. JAMA, Dec 4, 1996.

Grodstein F. Lancet 348:983–87, 1996.

Guarneri P, Guarneri R, Cascio C, Piccoli F, Papadopoulos V. *Gamma-Aminobutyric acid type A/benzodiazepine receptors regulate rat retina neurosteroidogenesis.* Brain Research 683 (1):65–72, 1995.

Guth L, Zhang A, Roberts E. *Key role for pregnenolone in combination therapy that promotes recovery after spinal cord injury.* Proceedings Nat Acad Sci of USA. 91(25): 12308–12, 1994.

Hammond G, Kontturi M, Vihko P, Vihko R. *Serum steroids in normal males and patients with prostatic disease.* Clin Endocrinol (oxf) 9(2): 113–21, 1978.

Harel Z, et al. *Supplementation with omega-3 polyunsaturated fatty acids in the management of dysmenorrhea in adolescents.* Am J Gynecol 174:1335–38, 1996.

Henderson E, Weinberg M, Wright W. *Pregnenolone.* J Clin Endcrinol 10:455–74, 1950.

Hoagland H. *Adventures in biological engineering.* Science 100: 63– 67, 1944.

Isaacson R, Varner J. *The effects of pregnenolone sulfate and ethylestrenol on retention of a passive avaoidance task.* Brain Res 689:79 –84, 1995.

JAMA 277(2):103, 1997.

Kavaliers M, Kinsella D. *Male preference for the odors of estrous female mice is reduced by the neurosteroid pregnenolone sulfate.* Brain Res 682:222–26, 1995. "Administration of Preg-S decreased male preference for the odors of estrous females, causing a significant dose-related (0.01-10 mg/kg) decrease in the amount of time spent in the proximity of the odors of the estrous female, while having significantly less of an effect on the responses to the non-estrous female odors. The effects of Preg-S were significantly reduced by peripheral administrations of the non-competitive NMDA receptor antagonist, MK-801, but were not significantly affected by either the GABAA antagonists, bicuculline and picrotoxin, or the benzodiazepine antagonist, Ro 15-1788. These results suggest that Preg-S has inhibitory effects on olfactory mediated male sexual interest, preference, or 'motivation' that, in part, involve interactions with NMDA receptor mediated mechanisms."

Koenig H, Schumacher M, Ferzaz B, Thi A, et al. *Progesterone synthesis and myelin formation by Schwann cells.* Science 268 (5216):1500 –03, 1995.

Lanthier A, Patwardhan V. *Sex steroids and 5-en-3-Beta-hydroxysteroids in specific regions of the human brain and cranial nerves.* J Steroid Biochem 25: 445– 49, 1986.

Maione S, Berrino L, Viagliano S, Leyva J, Rossi F. *Pregnenolone sulfate increases the convulsant potency of NMDA in mice.* Eur J Pharmacol 219(3):477 –79, 1992.

Majewska M. Bluet-Pajot M, Robel P, Baulieu E. *Pregnenlone sulfate antagonizes barbiturate-induced hypnosis.* Pharmacol Biochem Behav 33:(3):701–03, 1989.

Majewska M. *Neurosteroids: endogenous bimodal modulators of the GABA-A receptor: mechanism of action and physiological significance.* Progress in Neurobiology 38:379–95, 1992.

McGavack T, Chevalley J, Weissberg J. *The use of pregnenolone in various clinical disorders.* J Clin Endocrinol 11: 559–77, 1951.

Melchior CL, Ritzmann R. *Pregnenolone and pregnenolone sulfate, alone and with ethanol, in mice on the plus maze.* Pharmacol Biochem Behav 48:893–97, 1994.

Melchior CL, Ritzmann R. *Neurosteroids block the memory-impairing effects of ethanol in mice.* Pharmacol Biochem Behav, 53:51–56, 1996.

Morfin R, Young J, Corpechot C, Egestad B, Sjovall J, Baulieu E. *Neurosteroids: pregnenolone in human sciatic nerves.* Proc Natl Acad Sci USA 89(15):6790–93, 1992.

Notelovitz M. Modern Medicine 64:9–10, 1996.

Pincus G, Hoagland H. *Effects of administered pregnenolone on fatiguing psychomotor performance.* J Aviation Med 15: 98–115, 1944.

Pincus G, Hoagland H. *Effects on industrial production of the administration of pregnenolone to factory workers.* Psychosom Med 7: 342–46, 1945.

Ploeckinger B. British Med J 313:664, 1996.

Robel P, Baulieu, E. *DHEA is a neuroactive neurosteroid.* Ann NY Acad Sci 774:82–109, 1995.

Roberts E. *Pregnenolone—from Selye to Alzheimer and a model of the pregnenolone sulfate binding site on the GABA receptor.* Biochemical Pharmacology 49:1–16, 1995.

Roberts E, Faublet TJ. *Oral DHEA in MS.* In *The Biological Role of DHEA*, 1990. Kalimi M, Rogelson W, editors.

Romeo E, Brancati A, et al. *Marked decrease of plasma neuroactive steroids during alcohol withdrawal.* Clinical Neuropharmacology 19:366–69, 1996.

Selye H, Clarke E. *Potentiation of a pituitary extract with pregnenolone and additional observations concerning the influence of various organs on steroid metabolism.* Rev Can Biol 2:319–28, 1943.

Spiegel E, Wycis H. *Anticonvulsant effects of steroids.* J Lab & Clin Med 30:947–52, 1945.

Steiger A, Trachsel L, Guldner J. *Neurosteroid pregnenolone induces sleep-EEG changes in man compatible with inverse agonistic GABA receptor modulation.* Brain Res 615:267–74, 1993.

Sternberg T, LeVan P, Wright E. *The hydrating effects of pregnenolone acetate on the human skin.* Current Ther Res 3:11, 1961.

Stocco D, Clark B. *Role of the steroidogenic acute regulatory protein (StAR) in steroidogenesis.* Biochem Pharmacol 9, 51(3):197–205, 1992.

Tyler E, Payne S, Kirsch H. *Pregnenolone in male infertility.* West J Surg 56: 459–63, 1943.

Wang D, Bulbrook R, Ellis F, Coombs M. *Metabolic clearance rates of pregnenolone, 17-acetoxypregnenolone and their sulphate esters in man and in rabbit.* J Endocrinol 39:395–403, 1967.

Warner M, Gustafsson J. *Cytochrome P450 in the brain: neu-*

roendocrine functions. Front Neuroendocrinol 16(3): 224–36, 1995. "The effectiveness of steroid hormone metabolites as sedatives and anesthetics has been known for many years. More recently, their interaction with neurotransmitter receptors has helped to elucidate their mechanism of action, but their physiological functions and their role in disturbances of behavior, anxiety, and sleep/wakefulness have yet to be elucidated. Until 1981 it was assumed that metabolites of steroid hormones arose from the adrenals and gonads and that their action on neurotransmitter receptors was a mechanism of communication between the brain and the periphery. The evidence that the brain could accumulate steroids independently of the adrenals and gonads in 1981 and later the evidence for the presence of the cholesterol side chain cleavage enzyme (P450scc) in the brain have challenged this concept and stimulated a great deal of interest in the possibility that the brain could be making its own steroids from cholesterol for some as yet undefined purpose."

Wu F, Gibbs T, Farb D. *Pregnenolone sulfate: a positive allosteric modulator at the N-methyl-D-aspartate receptor.* Mol Pharmacol 40: 333–36, 1991.

Zumoff B, Strain G, Miller L, Rosner W. *Twenty-four hour mean plasma testosterone concentration declines wth age in nomal premenopausal women.* J Clin Endocrinol Metab 80: 1429–30. 1995.

Zureik M. British Med J 313:3–19, 1996.

Books

Current Medical Diagnosis and Treatment, 36th Edition, 1997. Tierney L, McPhee S, Papadakis M, editors. Appleton and Lange, publishers.

Principles of Ambulatory Medicine, 3rd Edition, 1991. Barker LR, Bunton Jr, Zieve PD, editors. Williams and Wilkins, publishers.

ABOUT THE AUTHOR

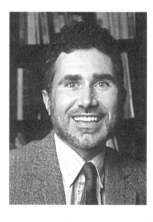

Ray Sahelian, M.D., is a physician certified by the American Board of Family Practice. He obtained a Bachelor of Science degree in nutrition from Drexel University and completed his doctoral training at Thomas Jefferson Medical School, both in Philadelphia. Following graduation he worked for three years as a resident in family medicine at Montgomery Hospital in Norristown, PA, and was involved with all aspects of medical care, including pediatrics, cardiology, obstetrics, oncology, psychiatry, and surgery.

A popular and respected physician and medical writer, Dr. Sahelian is internationally recognized as a moderate voice in the evaluation of leading-edge nutrients and hormones. He has been seen on numerous television programs including *CNN Talk Live*, *The Geraldo*

Rivera Show, The Maury Povich Show, A Current Affair, Extra, Dini Petty Show (Canada), and *Zone Interdite* (France); mentioned by countless major magazines such as *Newsweek, US News and World Report, Cosmopolitan, Modern Medicine, Health,* and *Internal Medicine News;* and quoted in hundreds of newspapers including *USA Today, The Los Angeles Times, The Washington Post, The Miami Herald, The Denver Post, Le Monde* (France), and *Que Pasa* (Chile). His articles have appeared in *Let's Live, Total Health, Healthy and Natural,* and others. Millions of listeners from over 1,000 radio stations nationwide have heard him discuss the latest research on hormones and nutrients.

Dr. Sahelian is the Editor of *Longevity Research Update,* and a nationally-known lecturer. He is also the author of the highly acclaimed *Be Happier Starting Now,* the best-selling *Melatonin: Nature's Sleeping Pill,* and *DHEA: A Practical Guide.* In addition, he is the coauthor of *Creatine: Nature's Muscle Builder.*

INDEX

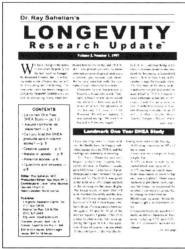

Research in hormone replacement therapy, nutrition, and longevity is accelerating. If you wish to keep up with the very latest information on melatonin, DHEA, pregnenolone, estrogen, progesterone, testosterone, growth hormone, other hormones, creatine, glucosamine, and other supplements, then this is the right newsletter for you. Dr. Sahelian and his staff constantly scan hundreds of new articles published in prestigious journals all over the world and present a balanced interpretation of the important findings. No hype, just the facts. We also discuss advances in the field of anti-aging science and how these advances can be practically applied to improve the quality of our lives.

8-page newsletter

The newsletter includes interviews with top experts, personal stories of hormone/supplement users, and a question-and-answer column. It is published in January, April, July, and October for 1996 and 1997. Beginning in 1998, the newsletter will be published six times a year, in January, March, May, July, September, and November. This newsletter was previously known as *Melatonin, DHEA, and Longevity Update.*

Self-Improvement and Success Books

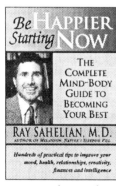

ISBN 09-639755-6-0
200 pages $12.00
© 1994, updated 1995

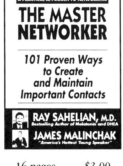

16 pages $3.00
© 1997

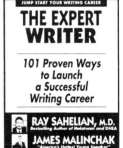

16 pages $3.00
© 1997

not available in stores

PLUS A REPORT ON
CHONDROITIN

GLUCOSAMINE

Nature's Arthritis Remedy

Includes the **latest research** on **diet, supplements,** and **hormones** that help relieve arthritic aches and pains.

RAY SAHELIAN, M.D.
Best-selling Author of Melatonin, DHEA, and Creatine and Editor of Longevity Research Update

26 pages $3.95
ISBN 0-9639755-2-8
© 1997

A DETAILED LOOK AT THE USE OF CREATINE

CREATINE
Nature's Muscle Builder

- ADDS STRENGTH AND POWER
- BUILDS LEAN MUSCLE MASS
- BOOSTS SPORTS ENDURANCE
- HELPS REDUCE BODY FAT

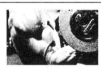

RAY SAHELIAN, M.D.
BESTSELLING AUTHOR OF MELATONIN AND DHEA
DAVE TUTTLE

144 pages $9.95
ISBN 0-89529-777-9
© 1997

More than 700,000 copies in print!

WHAT YOU NEED TO KNOW ABOUT DHEA

DHEA
A Practical Guide

THE NATURAL HORMONE THAT...

- HELPS FIGHT DISEASE
- IMPROVES MOOD & ENERGY
- BOOSTS YOUR SEX DRIVE
- INFLUENCES LONGEVITY

INCLUDES INTERVIEWS WITH THE WORLD'S TOP TWENTY DHEA RESEARCHERS

RAY SAHELIAN, M.D.
Bestselling Author of Melatonin: Nature's Sleeping Pill and Editor of Melatonin, DHEA, & Longevity Update

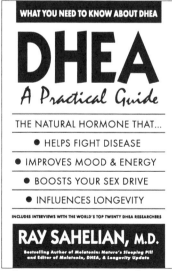

160 pages $9.95
ISBN 0-89529-774-4
© 1996, updated 1997

OVER 100,000 COPIES IN PRINT

MELATONIN
Nature's Sleeping Pill

THE NATURAL HORMONE THAT...

- RELIEVES INSOMNIA
- IMPROVES MOOD & ENERGY
- HELPS FIGHT DISEASE
- INFLUENCES LONGEVITY
- PREVENTS JET LAG

RAY SAHELIAN, M.D.
Bestselling Author of DHEA: A Practical Guide and Editor of Melatonin, DHEA, & Longevity Update

140 pages $9.95
ISBN 0-89529-775-2
© 1995, updated 1996

See web site **http://www.raysahelian.com** for latest updates.
To order by credit card call **310-821-2409** (best times are 9:00 a.m. to 5:00 p.m. Pacific Time, Monday through Friday) or copy/tear this page and mail in your order.

Name:_____

Address: _____

City/State/Zip:_____

Telephone: _____ E-mail:_____

Health Books and Newsletter

___ copies *Melatonin: Nature's Sleeping Pill* $ 9.95 _____

___ copies *DHEA: A Practical Guide* $ 9.95 _____

___ copies *Creatine: Nature's Muscle Builder* $ 9.95 _____

___ copies *Pregnenolone: Nature's Feel Good Hormone* $ 9.95 _____

___ copies *Glucosamine: Nature's Arthritis Remedy* $ 3.95 _____

❑   6 issues of *Longevity Research Update* $21.00 _____

❑   12 issues of *Longevity Research Update* $36.00 _____

❑   24 issues of *Longevity Research Update* $60.00 _____

Newsletters are published quarterly (January, April, July, October) in 1996 and 1997, and bimonthly starting in 1998.

___ Back issues of *Longevity Research Update* ($2.00 each)   _____

Self-Improvement and Success Books (great gift ideas!)

___ copies *Be Happier Starting Now* $12.00 _____

___ copies *The Master Networker* $ 3.00 _____

___ copies *The Expert Writer* $ 3.00 _____

No shipping charge for books mailed to US or Canada.
Shipping (airmail) for overseas: add $7.00 for first book, $4.00 for each additional book, and $0.70 for each newsletter.   _____

Tax on books shipped to California addresses is 8%   _____

Total: $_____

Books and newsletters are shipped promptly.
Twenty percent discount for 6 to 10 copies.
Thirty percent 11 to 15. Call for wholesale discount rate.

Please send a check for the total amount to:
Longevity Research Center, Inc.
P. O. Box 12619
Marina Del Rey, CA 90295

Credit Card # _____ Exp._____

We accept Visa, MC, AE, Diners Club, Carte Blanche, and JCB.